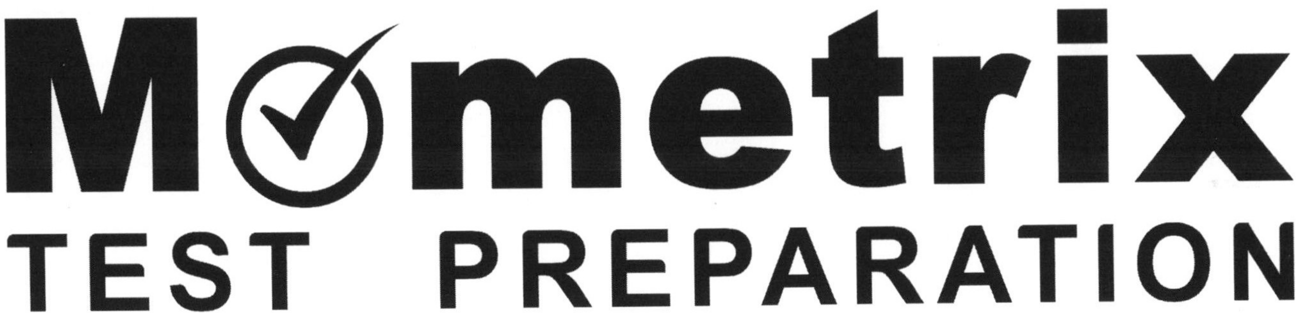

AF598775

Occupational Therapy Assistant Exam Secrets Study Guide

NBCOT®, COTA®, and Certified Occupational Therapy Assistant® are registered trademarks of the National Board for Certification in Occupational Therapy, Inc., which administers the NBCOT® exam. NBCOT does not endorse and is not affiliated in any way with Mometrix or its products and services.

Dear Future Exam Success Story

First of all, **THANK YOU** for purchasing Mometrix study materials!

Second, congratulations! You are one of the few determined test-takers who are committed to doing whatever it takes to excel on your exam. **You have come to the right place.** We developed these study materials with one goal in mind: to deliver you the information you need in a format that's concise and easy to use.

In addition to optimizing your guide for the content of the test, we've outlined our recommended steps for breaking down the preparation process into small, attainable goals so you can make sure you stay on track.

We've also analyzed the entire test-taking process, identifying the most common pitfalls and showing how you can overcome them and be ready for any curveball the test throws you.

Standardized testing is one of the biggest obstacles on your road to success, which only increases the importance of doing well in the high-pressure, high-stakes environment of test day. Your results on this test could have a significant impact on your future, and this guide provides the information and practical advice to help you achieve your full potential on test day.

Your success is our success

We would love to hear from you! If you would like to share the story of your exam success or if you have any questions or comments in regard to our products, please contact us at **800-673-8175** or **support@mometrix.com**.

Thanks again for your business and we wish you continued success!

Sincerely,
The Mometrix Test Preparation Team

Need more help? Check out our flashcards at:
http://mometrixflashcards.com/NBCOT

Copyright © 2026 by Mometrix Media LLC. All rights reserved.
Written and edited by the Mometrix Exam Secrets Test Prep Team
Printed in the United States of America

TABLE OF CONTENTS

Introduction

Thank you for purchasing this resource! You have made the choice to prepare yourself for a test that could have a huge impact on your future, and this guide is designed to help you be fully ready for test day. Obviously, it's important to have a solid understanding of the test material, but you also need to be prepared for the unique environment and stressors of the test, so that you can perform to the best of your abilities.

For this purpose, the first section that appears in this guide is the **Secret Keys**. We've devoted countless hours to meticulously researching what works and what doesn't, and we've boiled down our findings to the five most impactful steps you can take to improve your performance on the test. We start at the beginning with study planning and move through the preparation process, all the way to the testing strategies that will help you get the most out of what you know when you're finally sitting in front of the test.

We recommend that you start preparing for your test as far in advance as possible. However, if you've bought this guide as a last-minute study resource and only have a few days before your test, we recommend that you skip over the first two Secret Keys since they address a long-term study plan.

If you struggle with **test anxiety**, we strongly encourage you to check out our recommendations for how you can overcome it. Test anxiety is a formidable foe, but it can be beaten, and we want to make sure you have the tools you need to defeat it.

Copyright © Mometrix Media. You have been licensed one copy of this document for personal use only. Any other reproduction or redistribution is strictly prohibited. All rights reserved.
This content is provided for test preparation purposes only and does not imply an endorsement by Mometrix of any particular political, scientific, or religious point of view.

Secret Key #1 – Plan Big, Study Small

There's a lot riding on your performance. If you want to ace this test, you're going to need to keep your skills sharp and the material fresh in your mind. You need a plan that lets you review everything you need to know while still fitting in your schedule. We'll break this strategy down into three categories.

Information Organization

Start with the information you already have: the official test outline. From this, you can make a complete list of all the concepts you need to cover before the test. Organize these concepts into groups that can be studied together, and create a list of any related vocabulary you need to learn so you can brush up on any difficult terms. You'll want to keep this vocabulary list handy once you actually start studying since you may need to add to it along the way.

Time Management

Once you have your set of study concepts, decide how to spread them out over the time you have left before the test. Break your study plan into small, clear goals so you have a manageable task for each day and know exactly what you're doing. Then just focus on one small step at a time. When you manage your time this way, you don't need to spend hours at a time studying. Studying a small block of content for a short period each day helps you retain information better and avoid stressing over how much you have left to do. You can relax knowing that you have a plan to cover everything in time. In order for this strategy to be effective though, you have to start studying early and stick to your schedule. Avoid the exhaustion and futility that comes from last-minute cramming!

Study Environment

The environment you study in has a big impact on your learning. Studying in a coffee shop, while probably more enjoyable, is not likely to be as fruitful as studying in a quiet room. It's important to keep distractions to a minimum. You're only planning to study for a short block of time, so make the most of it. Don't pause to check your phone or get up to find a snack. It's also important to **avoid multitasking**. Research has consistently shown that multitasking will make your studying dramatically less effective. Your study area should also be comfortable and well-lit so you don't have the distraction of straining your eyes or sitting on an uncomfortable chair.

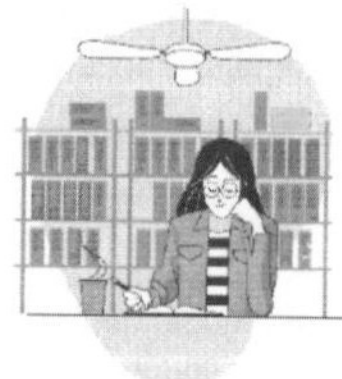

The time of day you study is also important. You want to be rested and alert. Don't wait until just before bedtime. Study when you'll be most likely to comprehend and remember. Even better, if you know what time of day your test will be, set that time aside for study. That way your brain will be used to working on that subject at that specific time and you'll have a better chance of recalling information.

Finally, it can be helpful to team up with others who are studying for the same test. Your actual studying should be done in as isolated an environment as possible, but the work of organizing the information and setting up the study plan can be divided up. In between study sessions, you can discuss with your teammates the concepts that you're all studying and quiz each other on the details. Just be sure that your teammates are as serious about the test as you are. If you find that your study time is being replaced with social time, you might need to find a new team.

Copyright © Mometrix Media. You have been licensed one copy of this document for personal use only. Any other reproduction or redistribution is strictly prohibited. All rights reserved.
This content is provided for test preparation purposes only and does not imply an endorsement by Mometrix of any particular political, scientific, or religious point of view.

Secret Key #2 – Make Your Studying Count

You're devoting a lot of time and effort to preparing for this test, so you want to be absolutely certain it will pay off. This means doing more than just reading the content and hoping you can remember it on test day. It's important to make every minute of study count. There are two main areas you can focus on to make your studying count.

Retention

It doesn't matter how much time you study if you can't remember the material. You need to make sure you are retaining the concepts. To check your retention of the information you're learning, try recalling it at later times with minimal prompting. Try carrying around flashcards and glance at one or two from time to time or ask a friend who's also studying for the test to quiz you.

To enhance your retention, look for ways to put the information into practice so that you can apply it rather than simply recalling it. If you're using the information in practical ways, it will be much easier to remember. Similarly, it helps to solidify a concept in your mind if you're not only reading it to yourself but also explaining it to someone else. Ask a friend to let you teach them about a concept you're a little shaky on (or speak aloud to an imaginary audience if necessary). As you try to summarize, define, give examples, and answer your friend's questions, you'll understand the concepts better and they will stay with you longer. Finally, step back for a big picture view and ask yourself how each piece of information fits with the whole subject. When you link the different concepts together and see them working together as a whole, it's easier to remember the individual components.

Finally, practice showing your work on any multi-step problems, even if you're just studying. Writing out each step you take to solve a problem will help solidify the process in your mind, and you'll be more likely to remember it during the test.

Modality

Modality simply refers to the means or method by which you study. Choosing a study modality that fits your own individual learning style is crucial. No two people learn best in exactly the same way, so it's important to know your strengths and use them to your advantage.

For example, if you learn best by visualization, focus on visualizing a concept in your mind and draw an image or a diagram. Try color-coding your notes, illustrating them, or creating symbols that will trigger your mind to recall a learned concept. If you learn best by hearing or discussing information, find a study partner who learns the same way or read aloud to yourself. Think about how to put the information in your own words. Imagine that you are giving a lecture on the topic and record yourself so you can listen to it later.

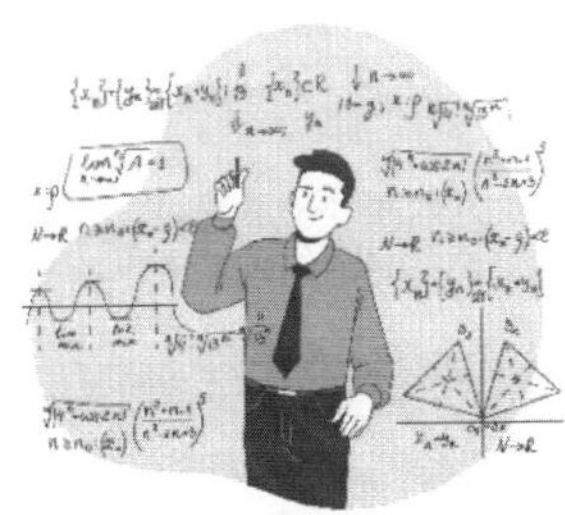

For any learning style, flashcards can be helpful. Organize the information so you can take advantage of spare moments to review. Underline key words or phrases. Use different colors for different categories. Mnemonic devices (such as creating a short list in which every item starts with the same letter) can also help with retention. Find what works best for you and use it to store the information in your mind most effectively and easily.

Copyright © Mometrix Media. You have been licensed one copy of this document for personal use only. Any other reproduction or redistribution is strictly prohibited. All rights reserved.
This content is provided for test preparation purposes only and does not imply an endorsement by Mometrix of any particular political, scientific, or religious point of view.

Secret Key #3 – Practice the Right Way

Your success on test day depends not only on how many hours you put into preparing, but also on whether you prepared the right way. It's good to check along the way to see if your studying is paying off. One of the most effective ways to do this is by taking practice tests to evaluate your progress. Practice tests are useful because they show exactly where you need to improve. Every time you take a practice test, pay special attention to these three groups of questions:

- The questions you got wrong
- The questions you had to guess on, even if you guessed right
- The questions you found difficult or slow to work through

This will show you exactly what your weak areas are, and where you need to devote more study time. Ask yourself why each of these questions gave you trouble. Was it because you didn't understand the material? Was it because you didn't remember the vocabulary? Do you need more repetitions on this type of question to build speed and confidence? Dig into those questions and figure out how you can strengthen your weak areas as you go back to review the material.

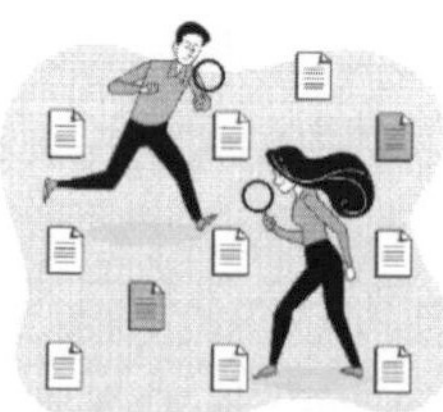

Additionally, many practice tests have a section explaining the answer choices. It can be tempting to read the explanation and think that you now have a good understanding of the concept. However, an explanation likely only covers part of the question's broader context. Even if the explanation makes perfect sense, **go back and investigate** every concept related to the question until you're positive you have a thorough understanding.

As you go along, keep in mind that the practice test is just that: practice. Memorizing these questions and answers will not be very helpful on the actual test because it is unlikely to have any of the same exact questions. If you only know the right answers to the sample questions, you won't be prepared for the real thing. **Study the concepts** until you understand them fully, and then you'll be able to answer any question that shows up on the test.

It's important to wait on the practice tests until you're ready. If you take a test on your first day of study, you may be overwhelmed by the amount of material covered and how much you need to learn. Work up to it gradually.

On test day, you'll need to be prepared for answering questions, managing your time, and using the test-taking strategies you've learned. It's a lot to balance, like a mental marathon that will have a big impact on your future. Like training for a marathon, you'll need to start slowly and work your way up. When test day arrives, you'll be ready.

Start with the strategies you've read in the first two Secret Keys—plan your course and study in the way that works best for you. If you have time, consider using multiple study resources to get different approaches to the same concepts. It can be helpful to see difficult concepts from more than one angle. Then find a good source for practice tests. Many times, the test website will suggest potential study resources or provide sample tests.

Copyright © Mometrix Media. You have been licensed one copy of this document for personal use only. Any other reproduction or redistribution is strictly prohibited. All rights reserved.
This content is provided for test preparation purposes only and does not imply an endorsement by Mometrix of any particular political, scientific, or religious point of view.

Practice Test Strategy

If you're able to find at least three practice tests, we recommend this strategy:

Untimed and Open-Book Practice

Take the first test with no time constraints and with your notes and study guide handy. Take your time and focus on applying the strategies you've learned.

Timed and Open-Book Practice

Take the second practice test open-book as well, but set a timer and practice pacing yourself to finish in time.

Timed and Closed-Book Practice

Take any other practice tests as if it were test day. Set a timer and put away your study materials. Sit at a table or desk in a quiet room, imagine yourself at the testing center, and answer questions as quickly and accurately as possible.

Keep repeating timed and closed-book tests on a regular basis until you run out of practice tests or it's time for the actual test. Your mind will be ready for the schedule and stress of test day, and you'll be able to focus on recalling the material you've learned.

Copyright © Mometrix Media. You have been licensed one copy of this document for personal use only. Any other reproduction or redistribution is strictly prohibited. All rights reserved.
This content is provided for test preparation purposes only and does not imply an endorsement by Mometrix of any particular political, scientific, or religious point of view.

Secret Key #4 – Pace Yourself

Once you're fully prepared for the material on the test, your biggest challenge on test day will be managing your time. Just knowing that the clock is ticking can make you panic even if you have plenty of time left. Work on pacing yourself so you can build confidence against the time constraints of the exam. Pacing is a difficult skill to master, especially in a high-pressure environment, so **practice is vital**.

Set time expectations for your pace based on how much time is available. For example, if a section has 60 questions and the time limit is 30 minutes, you know you have to average 30 seconds or less per question in order to answer them all. Although 30 seconds is the hard limit, set 25 seconds per question as your goal, so you reserve extra time to spend on harder questions. When you budget extra time for the harder questions, you no longer have any reason to stress when those questions take longer to answer.

Don't let this time expectation distract you from working through the test at a calm, steady pace, but keep it in mind so you don't spend too much time on any one question. Recognize that taking extra time on one question you don't understand may keep you from answering two that you do understand later in the test. If your time limit for a question is up and you're still not sure of the answer, mark it and move on, and come back to it later if the time and the test format allow. If the testing format doesn't allow you to return to earlier questions, just make an educated guess; then put it out of your mind and move on.

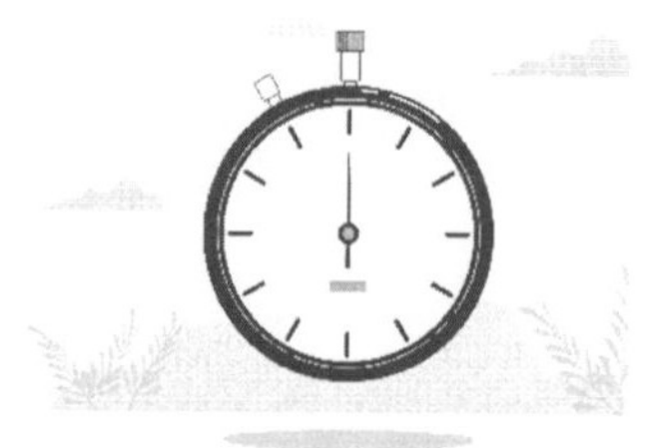

On the easier questions, be careful not to rush. It may seem wise to hurry through them so you have more time for the challenging ones, but it's not worth missing one if you know the concept and just didn't take the time to read the question fully. Work efficiently but make sure you understand the question and have looked at all of the answer choices, since more than one may seem right at first.

Even if you're paying attention to the time, you may find yourself a little behind at some point. You should speed up to get back on track, but do so wisely. Don't panic; just take a few seconds less on each question until you're caught up. Don't guess without thinking, but do look through the answer choices and eliminate any you know are wrong. If you can get down to two choices, it is often worthwhile to guess from those. Once you've chosen an answer, move on and don't dwell on any that you skipped or had to hurry through. If a question was taking too long, chances are it was one of the harder ones, so you weren't as likely to get it right anyway.

On the other hand, if you find yourself getting ahead of schedule, it may be beneficial to slow down a little. The more quickly you work, the more likely you are to make a careless mistake that will affect your score. You've budgeted time for each question, so don't be afraid to spend that time. Practice an efficient but careful pace to get the most out of the time you have.

Copyright © Mometrix Media. You have been licensed one copy of this document for personal use only. Any other reproduction or redistribution is strictly prohibited. All rights reserved.
This content is provided for test preparation purposes only and does not imply an endorsement by Mometrix of any particular political, scientific, or religious point of view.

Secret Key #5 – Have a Plan for Guessing

When you're taking the test, you may find yourself stuck on a question. Some of the answer choices seem better than others, but you don't see the one answer choice that is obviously correct. What do you do?

The scenario described above is very common, yet most test takers have not effectively prepared for it. Developing and practicing a plan for guessing may be one of the single most effective uses of your time as you get ready for the exam.

In developing your plan for guessing, there are three questions to address:

- When should you start the guessing process?
- How should you narrow down the choices?
- Which answer should you choose?

When to Start the Guessing Process

Unless your plan for guessing is to select C every time (which, despite its merits, is not what we recommend), you need to leave yourself enough time to apply your answer elimination strategies. Since you have a limited amount of time for each question, that means that if you're going to give yourself the best shot at guessing correctly, you have to decide quickly whether or not you will guess.

Of course, the best-case scenario is that you don't have to guess at all, so first, see if you can answer the question based on your knowledge of the subject and basic reasoning skills. Focus on the key words in the question and try to jog your memory of related topics. Give yourself a chance to bring the knowledge to mind, but once you realize that you don't have (or you can't access) the knowledge you need to answer the question, it's time to start the guessing process.

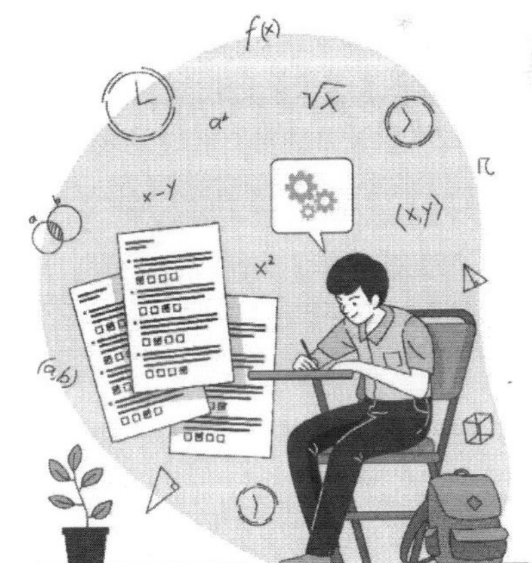

It's almost always better to start the guessing process too early than too late. It only takes a few seconds to remember something and answer the question from knowledge. Carefully eliminating wrong answer choices takes longer. Plus, going through the process of eliminating answer choices can actually help jog your memory.

Summary: Start the guessing process as soon as you decide that you can't answer the question based on your knowledge.

Copyright © Mometrix Media. You have been licensed one copy of this document for personal use only. Any other reproduction or redistribution is strictly prohibited. All rights reserved.
This content is provided for test preparation purposes only and does not imply an endorsement by Mometrix of any particular political, scientific, or religious point of view.

How to Narrow Down the Choices

The next chapter in this book (**Test-Taking Strategies**) includes a wide range of strategies for how to approach questions and how to look for answer choices to eliminate. You will definitely want to read those carefully, practice them, and figure out which ones work best for you. Here though, we're going to address a mindset rather than a particular strategy.

Your odds of guessing an answer correctly depend on how many options you are choosing from.

Number of options left	5	4	3	2	1
Odds of guessing correctly	20%	25%	33%	50%	100%

You can see from this chart just how valuable it is to be able to eliminate incorrect answers and make an educated guess, but there are two things that many test takers do that cause them to miss out on the benefits of guessing:

- Accidentally eliminating the correct answer
- Selecting an answer based on an impression

We'll look at the first one here, and the second one in the next section.

To avoid accidentally eliminating the correct answer, we recommend a thought exercise called **the $5 challenge**. In this challenge, you only eliminate an answer choice from contention if you are willing to bet $5 on it being wrong. Why $5? Five dollars is a small but not insignificant amount of money. It's an amount you could afford to lose but wouldn't want to throw away. And while losing $5 once might not hurt too much, doing it twenty times will set you back $100. In the same way, each small decision you make—eliminating a choice here, guessing on a question there—won't by itself impact your score very much, but when you put them all together, they can make a big difference. By holding each answer choice elimination decision to a higher standard, you can reduce the risk of accidentally eliminating the correct answer.

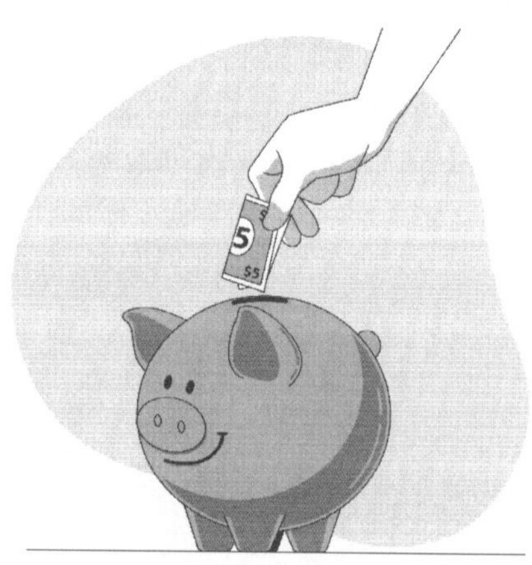

The $5 challenge can also be applied in a positive sense: If you are willing to bet $5 that an answer choice *is* correct, go ahead and mark it as correct.

Summary: Only eliminate an answer choice if you are willing to bet $5 that it is wrong.

Copyright © Mometrix Media. You have been licensed one copy of this document for personal use only. Any other reproduction or redistribution is strictly prohibited. All rights reserved.
This content is provided for test preparation purposes only and does not imply an endorsement by Mometrix of any particular political, scientific, or religious point of view.

Which Answer to Choose

You're taking the test. You've run into a hard question and decided you'll have to guess. You've eliminated all the answer choices you're willing to bet $5 on. Now you have to pick an answer. Why do we even need to talk about this? Why can't you just pick whichever one you feel like when the time comes?

The answer to these questions is that if you don't come into the test with a plan, you'll rely on your impression to select an answer choice, and if you do that, you risk falling into a trap. The test writers know that everyone who takes their test will be guessing on some of the questions, so they intentionally write wrong answer choices to seem plausible. You still have to pick an answer though, and if the wrong answer choices are designed to look right, how can you ever be sure that you're not falling for their trap? The best solution we've found to this dilemma is to take the decision out of your hands entirely. Here is the process we recommend:

Once you've eliminated any choices that you are confident (willing to bet $5) are wrong, select the first remaining choice as your answer.

Whether you choose to select the first remaining choice, the second, or the last, the important thing is that you use some preselected standard. Using this approach guarantees that you will not be enticed into selecting an answer choice that looks right, because you are not basing your decision on how the answer choices look.

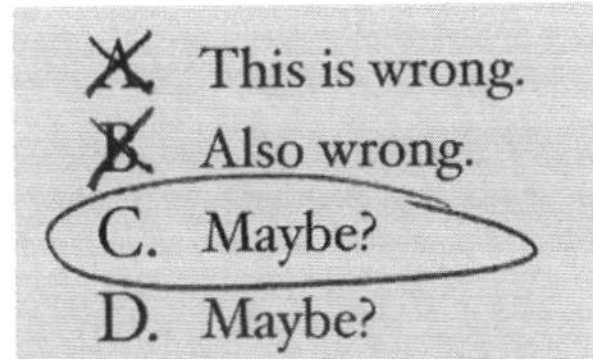

This is not meant to make you question your knowledge. Instead, it is to help you recognize the difference between your knowledge and your impressions. There's a huge difference between thinking an answer is right because of what you know, and thinking an answer is right because it looks or sounds like it should be right.

Summary: To ensure that your selection is appropriately random, make a predetermined selection from among all answer choices you have not eliminated.

Copyright © Mometrix Media. You have been licensed one copy of this document for personal use only. Any other reproduction or redistribution is strictly prohibited. All rights reserved.
This content is provided for test preparation purposes only and does not imply an endorsement by Mometrix of any particular political, scientific, or religious point of view.

Test-Taking Strategies

This section contains a list of test-taking strategies that you may find helpful as you work through the test. By taking what you know and applying logical thought, you can maximize your chances of answering any question correctly!

It is very important to realize that every question is different and every person is different: no single strategy will work on every question, and no single strategy will work for every person. That's why we've included all of them here, so you can try them out and determine which ones work best for different types of questions and which ones work best for you.

Question Strategies

☑ Read Carefully

Read the question and the answer choices carefully. Don't miss the question because you misread the terms. You have plenty of time to read each question thoroughly and make sure you understand what is being asked. Yet a happy medium must be attained, so don't waste too much time. You must read carefully and efficiently.

☑ Contextual Clues

Look for contextual clues. If the question includes a word you are not familiar with, look at the immediate context for some indication of what the word might mean. Contextual clues can often give you all the information you need to decipher the meaning of an unfamiliar word. Even if you can't determine the meaning, you may be able to narrow down the possibilities enough to make a solid guess at the answer to the question.

☑ Prefixes

If you're having trouble with a word in the question or answer choices, try dissecting it. Take advantage of every clue that the word might include. Prefixes can be a huge help. Usually, they allow you to determine a basic meaning. *Pre-* means before, *post-* means after, *pro-* is positive, *de-* is negative. From prefixes, you can get an idea of the general meaning of the word and try to put it into context.

☑ Hedge Words

Watch out for critical hedge words, such as *likely, may, can, often, almost, mostly, usually, generally, rarely,* and *sometimes.* Question writers insert these hedge phrases to cover every possibility. Often an answer choice will be wrong simply because it leaves no room for exception. Be on guard for answer choices that have definitive words such as *exactly* and *always.*

☑ Switchback Words

Stay alert for *switchbacks.* These are the words and phrases frequently used to alert you to shifts in thought. The most common switchback words are *but, although,* and *however.* Others include *nevertheless, on the other hand, even though, while, in spite of, despite,* and *regardless of.* Switchback words are important to catch because they can change the direction of the question or an answer choice.

Copyright © Mometrix Media. You have been licensed one copy of this document for personal use only. Any other reproduction or redistribution is strictly prohibited. All rights reserved.
This content is provided for test preparation purposes only and does not imply an endorsement by Mometrix of any particular political, scientific, or religious point of view.

✓ Face Value

When in doubt, use common sense. Accept the situation in the problem at face value. Don't read too much into it. These problems will not require you to make wild assumptions. If you have to go beyond creativity and warp time or space in order to have an answer choice fit the question, then you should move on and consider the other answer choices. These are normal problems rooted in reality. The applicable relationship or explanation may not be readily apparent, but it is there for you to figure out. Use your common sense to interpret anything that isn't clear.

Answer Choice Strategies

✓ Answer Selection

The most thorough way to pick an answer choice is to identify and eliminate wrong answers until only one is left, then confirm it is the correct answer. Sometimes an answer choice may immediately seem right, but be careful. The test writers will usually put more than one reasonable answer choice on each question, so take a second to read all of them and make sure that the other choices are not equally obvious. As long as you have time left, it is better to read every answer choice than to pick the first one that looks right without checking the others.

✓ Answer Choice Families

An answer choice family consists of two (in rare cases, three) answer choices that are very similar in construction and cannot all be true at the same time. If you see two answer choices that are direct opposites or parallels, one of them is usually the correct answer. For instance, if one answer choice says that quantity *x* increases and another either says that quantity *x* decreases (opposite) or says that quantity *y* increases (parallel), then those answer choices would fall into the same family. An answer choice that doesn't match the construction of the answer choice family is more likely to be incorrect. Most questions will not have answer choice families, but when they do appear, you should be prepared to recognize them.

✓ Eliminate Answers

Eliminate answer choices as soon as you realize they are wrong, but make sure you consider all possibilities. If you are eliminating answer choices and realize that the last one you are left with is also wrong, don't panic. Start over and consider each choice again. There may be something you missed the first time that you will realize on the second pass.

✓ Avoid Fact Traps

Don't be distracted by an answer choice that is factually true but doesn't answer the question. You are looking for the choice that answers the question. Stay focused on what the question is asking for so you don't accidentally pick an answer that is true but incorrect. Always go back to the question and make sure the answer choice you've selected actually answers the question and is not merely a true statement.

✓ Extreme Statements

In general, you should avoid answers that put forth extreme actions as standard practice or proclaim controversial ideas as established fact. An answer choice that states the "process should be used in certain situations, if..." is much more likely to be correct than one that states the "process should be discontinued completely." The first is a calm rational statement and doesn't even make a definitive, uncompromising stance, using a hedge word *if* to provide wiggle room, whereas the second choice is far more extreme.

Copyright © Mometrix Media. You have been licensed one copy of this document for personal use only. Any other reproduction or redistribution is strictly prohibited. All rights reserved.
This content is provided for test preparation purposes only and does not imply an endorsement by Mometrix of any particular political, scientific, or religious point of view.

✓ Benchmark

As you read through the answer choices and you come across one that seems to answer the question well, mentally select that answer choice. This is not your final answer, but it's the one that will help you evaluate the other answer choices. The one that you selected is your benchmark or standard for judging each of the other answer choices. Every other answer choice must be compared to your benchmark. That choice is correct until proven otherwise by another answer choice beating it. If you find a better answer, then that one becomes your new benchmark. Once you've decided that no other choice answers the question as well as your benchmark, you have your final answer.

✓ Predict the Answer

Before you even start looking at the answer choices, it is often best to try to predict the answer. When you come up with the answer on your own, it is easier to avoid distractions and traps because you will know exactly what to look for. The right answer choice is unlikely to be word-for-word what you came up with, but it should be a close match. Even if you are confident that you have the right answer, you should still take the time to read each option before moving on.

General Strategies

✓ Tough Questions

If you are stumped on a problem or it appears too hard or too difficult, don't waste time. Move on! Remember though, if you can quickly check for obviously incorrect answer choices, your chances of guessing correctly are greatly improved. Before you completely give up, at least try to knock out a couple of possible answers. Eliminate what you can and then guess at the remaining answer choices before moving on.

✓ Check Your Work

Since you will probably not know every term listed and the answer to every question, it is important that you get credit for the ones that you do know. Don't miss any questions through careless mistakes. If at all possible, try to take a second to look back over your answer selection and make sure you've selected the correct answer choice and haven't made a costly careless mistake (such as marking an answer choice that you didn't mean to mark). This quick double check should more than pay for itself in caught mistakes for the time it costs.

✓ Pace Yourself

It's easy to be overwhelmed when you're looking at a page full of questions; your mind is confused and full of random thoughts, and the clock is ticking down faster than you would like. Calm down and maintain the pace that you have set for yourself. Especially as you get down to the last few minutes of the test, don't let the small numbers on the clock make you panic. As long as you are on track by monitoring your pace, you are guaranteed to have time for each question.

✓ Don't Rush

It is very easy to make errors when you are in a hurry. Maintaining a fast pace in answering questions is pointless if it makes you miss questions that you would have gotten right otherwise. Test writers like to include distracting information and wrong answers that seem right. Taking a little extra time to avoid careless mistakes can make all the difference in your test score. Find a pace that allows you to be confident in the answers that you select.

Copyright © Mometrix Media. You have been licensed one copy of this document for personal use only. Any other reproduction or redistribution is strictly prohibited. All rights reserved.
This content is provided for test preparation purposes only and does not imply an endorsement by Mometrix of any particular political, scientific, or religious point of view.

☑ Keep Moving

Panicking will not help you pass the test, so do your best to stay calm and keep moving. Taking deep breaths and going through the answer elimination steps you practiced can help to break through a stress barrier and keep your pace.

Final Notes

The combination of a solid foundation of content knowledge and the confidence that comes from practicing your plan for applying that knowledge is the key to maximizing your performance on test day. As your foundation of content knowledge is built up and strengthened, you'll find that the strategies included in this chapter become more and more effective in helping you quickly sift through the distractions and traps of the test to isolate the correct answer.

Now that you're preparing to move forward into the test content chapters of this book, be sure to keep your goal in mind. As you read, think about how you will be able to apply this information on the test. If you've already seen sample questions for the test and you have an idea of the question format and style, try to come up with questions of your own that you can answer based on what you're reading. This will give you valuable practice applying your knowledge in the same ways you can expect to on test day.

Good luck and good studying!

Copyright © Mometrix Media. You have been licensed one copy of this document for personal use only. Any other reproduction or redistribution is strictly prohibited. All rights reserved.
This content is provided for test preparation purposes only and does not imply an endorsement by Mometrix of any particular political, scientific, or religious point of view.

Copyright © Mometrix Media. You have been licensed one copy of this document for personal use only. Any other reproduction or redistribution is strictly prohibited. All rights reserved.
This content is provided for test preparation purposes only and does not imply an endorsement by Mometrix of any particular political, scientific, or religious point of view.

Collaborating and Gathering Information

Factors that Impact Occupational Performance

Developmental Milestones for Ages 0–12 Months

From 0–6 months, the infant begins to develop mature hearing and can respond to sound. Sight becomes more acute also as the infant is beginning to be able to track objects. Coordinated movement is mainly in the form of sucking, swallowing, and rhythmical movements of tongue and jaw for feeding. From 6–12 months, the infant can begin to use hands in a coordinated movement to play with a single toy and imitate gestures. The infant is also able to move food around the mouth as well as begin to chew food. This is a time in which different texture foods are tolerated. Coordinated hand movements around mealtime focus on picking up finger foods and holding a cup. Finger foods are things like crackers. Holding a cup is often done with both hands and dual handles on the cup.

Development of Grasp from 4 Months to 3 Years Old

At 4 months, infants can approach an object and pull the object back toward them. No thumb movement is used. By 5 months, infants can place fingers on top of an object and press it into the center of the palm with the thumb adducted (palmar grasp). During the 6th month, objects are grasped with the thumb on the side of the object and the radial side of the palm and wrist straight (radial-palmar grasp). By month 8, an infant can hold an object with an opposed thumb and fingertips (radial-digital grasp). By 1 year of age, a baby can place an object between the fingertips and distal joints of the fingers (pincer grasp). Fisted grip in which an object is held in a palmar supinated grasp is developed usually by 1 ½ years. Finally, by 2-3 years of age, the wrist is in neutral with the forearm pronated while the arm moves as one unit.

Role of Exploration in a Child's Development

Part of being a child is to have an inquisitive mind with a willingness to explore the environment. However, autistic children have much anxiety when structure is decreased and exploration is encouraged. Exploration should begin with toys that are age appropriate. Choices for exploration are limited, at first, to not overwhelm the senses. As the child increases in curiosity and begins to indicate a readiness to explore, more choices are given and exploration encouraged. Like all therapy, the home program is very important as it continues to focus in a structured manner on exploration of the environment. Positive reinforcements are very important as they encourage the desired behavior by the child. Exploration is the way a child learns to crawl, walk, and run. All milestones involve some form of exploration. Keeping exploration fun for the child is key to a positive experience.

Rheumatoid Arthritis

Rheumatoid arthritis is a systemic condition affecting the autoimmune system. In rheumatoid arthritis, the joints in the hands, wrists, ankles, shoulders, and hips are affected with pain, stiffness, limited range of motion (ROM), swelling, and deformities. Hand deformities are in the form of Boutonniere and Swann neck deformities. A Boutonniere deformity is the flexion of proximal interphalangeal (PIP) and hyper-extension of DIP joints of the hands. A Swann neck deformity is hyper-extension of the PIP and flexion of the distal interphalangeal (DIP) joints. People with rheumatoid arthritis have difficulty with activities of daily living (ADLs) and instrumental activities of daily living (IADLs), such as donning or doffing clothing, buttoning and snapping clothing, cooking, cleaning, and performing any activities that requires lifting and fine motor skills.

Copyright © Mometrix Media. You have been licensed one copy of this document for personal use only. Any other reproduction or redistribution is strictly prohibited. All rights reserved.
This content is provided for test preparation purposes only and does not imply an endorsement by Mometrix of any particular political, scientific, or religious point of view.

Treatment often is focused on adaptive equipment to assist the patient to return to performing daily tasks.

Osteoarthritis

Osteoarthritis arthritis is a degenerative joint disease that occurs when cartilage breaks down and leads to pain, swelling, and stiffness. This form of arthritis occurs mainly in the hips, knees, back, neck, shoulders, elbows, and fingers. Symptoms are limited range of motion (ROM) and stiffness and clicking sound of the joint when the cartilage is worn as two bones rub together. Pain is often worse at the end of the day or after activity. The purpose of joint surgery is sometimes to replace worn joints of the hips and knees. Treatment focuses on pain relief through gentle exercise, ROM stretching, and heat. Osteoarthritis affects one's ability to perform activities of daily living (ADLs) as well as instrumental activities of daily living (IADLs). Treatment focuses on adaptive equipment, strengthening and increasing ROM, transfers, and functional mobility throughout the home to perform tasks safely. Often, the client is taught adaptive strategies to perform tasks in a manner that preserves remaining joint function.

Left Versus Right Hemispheric Stroke

Left hemispheric stokes occur on the left side of the brain but affect the right side of the body. These strokes tend to affect speech, language, and memory. Weakness can occur on the right side of the body. These types of strokes often cause aphasia—a language problem affecting the understanding of language as well as the ability to speak. In motor apraxia— the inability to perform purposeful movements as well as verbal apraxia—problems motorically forming words are often present with this type of stroke also. A right hemispheric stroke is associated with left motor damage. Right hemispheric strokes affect emotion, abstract meaning, organization, visual information, as well as memory. People with right hemispheric strokes often have left-sided neglect. People with right hemispheric strokes will often have problems with spatial relations as well as visual perceptual difficulties.

Carpal Tunnel Syndrome

Carpal tunnel is characterized as compression of the median nerve of the wrist as it passes through the volar side of the wrist. Symptoms of carpal tunnel are mainly numbness, tingling, and/or pain in the thumb, index, middle, and ring fingers. The causes of this syndrome are often repetitive motions such as typing, fine motor tasks, and any activity that involves repetitive motion of the wrist. Conservative treatment consists of rest as well as anti-inflammatory medication. Therapy involves splinting the wrist to immobilize the wrist flexors (especially during sleep). Nerve gliding exercises, strengthening, and education on activity changes to prevent further flare-ups are all part of the occupational therapy treatment for carpal tunnel. Surgical treatment is often endoscopic, with a small incision just below and above the carpal tunnel area of the volar wrist. Micro-surgery makes recovery and wound care simpler and faster.

Influence of Values, Beliefs, and Spirituality on Occupational Performance

Spirituality is an important part of many people's lives. Spirituality and beliefs are a part of most people's lives. Religious awareness as well as a belief system that includes a belief in a higher being have been shown to contribute to healing and the rehabilitative process. The extent to which clients prioritize the activities they want to return to doing after an illness is related to the value system that family, friends, and society places on returning to previous roles or learning new roles within the family, workplace, and society. Interestingly, spirituality has also been linked to the recovery process. Studies have shown that people with strong spiritual beliefs recover quicker from illness than those without deep-rooted beliefs.

Copyright © Mometrix Media. You have been licensed one copy of this document for personal use only. Any other reproduction or redistribution is strictly prohibited. All rights reserved.
This content is provided for test preparation purposes only and does not imply an endorsement by Mometrix of any particular political, scientific, or religious point of view.

Obtaining Information Relevant to an Occupational Profile

Chart Review

A thorough chart review is critical for obtaining objective medical information. Past medical history, history of present illness, precautions, current treatments, and medications are all important subjects to review prior to interviewing and examining the client. Past medical history can give insight into factors leading to the current illness as well as premorbid functional level. The course of the current illness is useful to determine acuity level as well as realistic short- and long-term goals. Precautions are important in determining which treatments should be avoided based upon current condition. Finally, medications are useful to review to know what side effects may affect participation in therapy.

Interviewing the Client

The client is one of the main sources of information. The client supplies information concerning their premorbid status. The therapist can get a full picture of the client's activity level from a chart review as well as an interview. Activities of daily living such as bathing, dressing, toileting, and grooming are useful for the occupational therapist. Transfers to the toilet, tub, or shower, as well as functional mobility in rooms of the home, clue the therapist to safety concerns such as balance, fall risk, and the need for adaptive equipment. Through the interview process, vocational and avocational interests are determined to obtain a complete understanding of activities performed outside of the home.

Interviewing Caregivers and Family Members

Family and caregivers are also part of the puzzle to figuring out premorbid status, history of illness, and goals for therapy. Many times, due to illness, the family may have a different viewpoint from the client when it comes to historical data. Due to cognitive decline and/or illness, patients often have cognitive deficits that affect recall. Thus, clients are sometimes poor historians and need the input of family members to complete the whole clinical picture for the therapist. The seasoned therapist will look for verbal as well as nonverbal cues. Many times, family members are reluctant to talk in front of the client. However, acute observation will reveal what is not said (through expressions and gestures) as well as what is said.

Observing Clients Perform Self-Care Tasks

Although a chart review and interviewing the client and family are all part of collecting background information, the assessment is when the therapist can observe the client perform activities of daily living as well as advanced tasks (i.e., cooking) to determine the short- and long-term goals for therapy. During observation, the therapist determines quality of movement, deficits, safety, and potential for rehab. Once observations are recorded and potential for rehab has been determined, goals can be set. Finally, observation serves to reconcile the difference between what is reported by the client and family and what is actually observed by the therapist.

Reviewing the Chart and Evaluation of OTR

The certified occupational therapy assistant (COTA) is responsible for reviewing the complete chart of the patient. This review should include past history and current history as well as the occupational therapist, registered (OTR) evaluation. Some therapists include a review of other disciplines' evaluation to adequately get the full medical picture of the client. The COTA should be cognizant of medications and their interactions with treatments such as exercise, precautions, and medical procedures. A review of new medical notes should take place on a daily basis with a thorough review of any OTR progress notes and reevaluations on a weekly basis. The COTA should be just as informed as the OTR as to the condition of the patient. As with the OTR, the COTA should

Copyright © Mometrix Media. You have been licensed one copy of this document for personal use only. Any other reproduction or redistribution is strictly prohibited. All rights reserved.
This content is provided for test preparation purposes only and does not imply an endorsement by Mometrix of any particular political, scientific, or religious point of view.

ask questions regarding any orders, precautions, or comments added to the medical chart that are not understood.

FACTORS IN CHOOSING AN ASSESSMENT DURING AN EVALUATION

An occupational therapist must determine several factors to perform the appropriate assessment. The assessment must relate to the context in which the assessment is intended (i.e., traumatic brain injury, spinal cord injury, safety following a stroke, home safety following a hip replacement, etc.). The primary setting the person lives as well as his or her roles, values, norms, and support are also important when considering an assessment. In context of the client, chronological and developmental age must be considered as well as the stage, length, and expected outcomes of the illness. Finally, the validity and reliability of the assessment must be considered.

STANDARD GONIOMETRIC MEASUREMENT

A goniometer is an instrument that measures angles. The goniometer is commonly used in occupational therapy to measure the range of motion of a joint in the body. This measurement allows the tracking of progress (increases in range of motion) during therapy sessions. Without this measurement, progress is subjective instead of objective. Knowledge of standard procedures for goniometry as well as knowledge of anatomy is essential to performing goniometry. This type of measurement is useful after orthopedic surgeries such as knee replacement, hip replacement, as well as other joint replacement and repair. Goniometry is not useful in cases in which there is no expectation of an increase in active range of motion or in cases in which increased tone influences range of motion. Examples in which you may choose not to use goniometry are stroke patients or those with a head injury or severe arthritis.

MANUAL MUSCLE TEST

A manual muscle test measures the contraction of a muscle. This is commonly used after an illness or injury to measure the effect of immobilization or the disease process on the strength of a muscle. This is important to identify the course of rehabilitation. A manual muscle test may be performed with gravity eliminated (usually side-lying) or against gravity (usually sitting or standing). If a muscle is unable to resist a push or pull against gravity, it is rated 2+/5 or less. If a muscle is able to resist a push or pull against gravity, it is rated 3/5 or better. The rating scale ranges from 0/5 for no strength to 5/5 for full strength. Protocol for the manual muscle test states to test the non-injured side first. Test with gravity eliminated and then against gravity. Stabilize unrelated proximal joints to prevent unnecessary muscle compensation.

INTERDISCIPLINARY METHODS WHEN STROKE VICTIM WANTS TO RETURN TO DRIVING

A stroke patient will frequently be unaware of his or her deficits. As part of the stroke, neglect of a visual field, side of body, and a change in visual perceptual abilities are common. Because driving involves attention to all visual fields, spatial awareness, awareness of both sides of the body, and the ability to compensate for deficits, each discipline should perform standardized testing that identifies deficits in these categories. An occupational therapist may perform tests for visual perceptual skills. Psychology may perform tests for judgment, memory, and attention. Speech therapy may test for language comprehension (verbal and nonverbal). Together, a determination can be made about how deficits affect the client and strategies to compensate for deficits. In some cases, compensatory techniques are appropriate. However, severe deficits may mean that driving is no longer safe for the client to perform.

SLUMS AND MMSE FOR COGNITIVE TESTING

The Saint Louis University Mental Status examination (SLUMS) examination asks questions related to orientation, short-term memory, calculation, figure differentiation, size differentiation, clock

Copyright © Mometrix Media. You have been licensed one copy of this document for personal use only. Any other reproduction or redistribution is strictly prohibited. All rights reserved.
This content is provided for test preparation purposes only and does not imply an endorsement by Mometrix of any particular political, scientific, or religious point of view.

orientation, and animal naming to assess orientation, memory, and executive functioning. The purpose of the SLUMS examination is to test mild cognitive impairment as well as dementia. The Mini-Mental State Examination (MMSE) is also a short cognitive test. This exam tests orientation, registration, attention, calculation, and language and praxis. The scores range from no cognitive impairment to cognitive impairment. These tools should not be used by themselves but in context to activities of daily living (ADL) and instrumental activities of daily living (IADL) assessments and other functional tests. This is especially true for the early stages of dementia as rote skills are often performed with the presence of slowly declining cognitive function. Skills such as ADLs often are affected in the middle and later stages of dementia.

FIM Assessment

The Functional Independence Measure (FIM) is used to assess the following skills: eating; grooming; bathing; upper body dressing; lower body dressing; toileting; bladder and bowel management; transfers to bed, wheelchair, toilet, and tub or shower; ambulation or wheelchair mobility; mobility up and down stairs; comprehension; expression; social interaction; problem-solving; and memory. Each item on the FIM is observed by the therapist and rated on a scale of 1–7. A score of 1 means the patient is totally dependent with the activity. A score of 2 means the person is able to perform less than 50% of the activity on his or her own. A score of 3 means the client is able to perform between 50% and 75% of the task. A score of 4 means the client requires less than 25% assistance. A score of 5 means the activity can be performed with supervision. A score of 6 means that the client is able to perform the task on his or her own but may need additional time to complete it. Finally, a score of 7 means the client is able to perform the task on his or her own, safely, and with no additional time.

Allen Cognitive Model

The Allen Cognitive Model is centered on cognition. This model involves the interaction between cognitive abilities and the activity setting. Both cognitive abilities and activity settings affect performance. There are seven levels of cognition: coma (0), awareness (1), gross body movements (2), manual actions (3), familiar activity (4), learning new activities (5), and planning new activities (6). The Allen Cognitive Model assists caregivers to assess a person's functional cognition. Once the client's cognitive level is identified, focus can begin on maximizing abilities with remaining cognitive skills. This is important in working with patients who have dementia. This model was designed not only for use by professional caregivers, such as occupational therapists but for use by family members who assist the client in daily tasks. By way of knowing what stage a client is demonstrating, appropriate interaction and goals can be achieved.

Fine Motor Coordination Assessment

Dexterity tests measure accuracy of hand and finger movements. There are several good assessments that can be used to test dexterity. The Minnesota manual dexterity test involves placing round pegs in a pegboard in a quick, timed fashion. This test can be used to assess carpal tunnel syndrome as well as other hand and wrist injuries. The box and block test use cubes and focus on picking up the cubes and placing them into a nearby container. The grooved pegboard test requires the client to placed grooved pins in a pegboard. The big difference in this test is that the client has to have enough dexterity to rotate the pin to the correct orientation so that it fits in the hole. Finally, the Purdue pegboard test uses both hands to respectively place pegs into the pegboard. Washers and collars are then placed over the pegs in a prescribed fashion.

Hand Strength Tests

A dynamometer is a device that the client squeezes with a hand to tell the strength of a grip. This test is usually performed by holding the dynamometer at a 90-degree bend of the elbow (with the

Copyright © Mometrix Media. You have been licensed one copy of this document for personal use only. Any other reproduction or redistribution is strictly prohibited. All rights reserved.
This content is provided for test preparation purposes only and does not imply an endorsement by Mometrix of any particular political, scientific, or religious point of view.

elbow to the side). The client then squeezes the dynamometer three times to ascertain muscle strength and endurance. The average of the three squeezes is the final score recorded. Finger strength is tested with a pinch meter. The three most common grips tested are lateral pinch, in which a pinch meter is placed between the pad of the thumb and the lateral surface of the index finger. The three-point pinch is performed by placing the pinch meter between the pad of the thumb and the pad of the index and middle fingers. Finally, two-point pinch is performed by placing the pinch meter between the tip of the thumb and the tip of the index finger.

Benefit of Performing On-Site Work or Home Evaluations

The clinic setting provides only a limited opportunity to perform analysis and treatment. Observations are made based on simulation. The client interview is important but, likewise, can account only for what can be described. The workplace evaluation and training allow the occupational therapist (OT) or occupational therapy assistant (OTA) to assess the client in his or her work environment. The actual work space as well as other requirements do not have to be simulated. Likewise, a home an assessment is better than simulation in a clinic as it offers the ability for the OT to observe the client in his or her own environment and determine, based upon the home environment, equipment and training needs. A checklist often forms the basis for the evaluation or training in this context. The checklist will contain the occupational components necessary to complete the task. The client is then graded based upon his or her ability to perform these components. Further treatments can then focus on deficits found in the home and/or workplace.

Internal Factors That Affect a Client's Engagement in Occupation

The sensory factors that affect a client's ability to engage in meaningful activity are related to vestibular functions, hearing functions, visual functions, taste functions, smell functions, proprioceptive functions, touch functions, pain, and sensitivity to temperature and pressure. Vestibular functions have to do with position, balance, and movement against gravity. Proprioceptive functions concern awareness of one's body position in space. All of the senses depend upon each other to form a complete sensory picture of the client's environment. Muscle functions work together with sensory functions to produce meaningful, controlled movement. Mental functions such as attention, memory, perception, emotion, and higher-level cognitive skills work together to form awareness. Finally, higher-level skills such as judgment, executive functions, praxis, and concept formation utilize a higher level of functioning and are useful for forming complex thoughts.

Influence of Habits and Routines on Meaningful Engagement

Habits are repetitive actions. These actions can be part of a daily routine or in response to certain stimuli. Most individuals have a favorite routine performed on a daily basis. Over time, these become habits. Habits are also reflective of values. In turn, personal values are often based upon the roles and routines expected within life, work, and recreation communities. The habits formed affect the occupations that are valued and pursued. Habits influence occupations at work, school, play, and home. Routines are the normal way of doing things in a particular order. For, instance a nighttime habit may be to drink a glass of milk before sleep. A routine may be the order of events prior to going to bed, for instance, showering, brushing teeth, getting into the bed, and then reading.

Relationship of Roles and Purposeful Activity

Individuals have roles within their family, work, and school environments. For instance, they may be a parent at home and a manager at work. Each requires a different set of skills or occupations. A parent may need to have perfected occupations such as being able to perform the instrumental activities of daily living (IADL) skills of yard work, housecleaning, and parenting. A manager, however, may need to perform occupations related to accounting, management, and computers.

Copyright © Mometrix Media. You have been licensed one copy of this document for personal use only. Any other reproduction or redistribution is strictly prohibited. All rights reserved.
This content is provided for test preparation purposes only and does not imply an endorsement by Mometrix of any particular political, scientific, or religious point of view.

Each of these roles requires skills that make meaningful engagement in family and work life. Although there are skills unique to each role, there are also overlapping skills. For instance, organizational skills are required of both a parent and manager. The overlapping of skills is not uncommon as many roles need basic skills such as decision-making, organizing, planning, controlling, and interpersonal and leadership abilities.

Role of OT in Mental Health Discharge Planning

Mental health has some unique issues that require special discharge planning for team and family members. Many of the issues surrounding discharge have to do with psychosocial concerns. The occupational therapist works with team members to adjust behaviors, coping skills, and thought processes of their clients. Follow-through in the home environment is essential for the patient and should be addressed with family members and caregivers prior to discharge. Support systems must be in place to ensure the patient does not regress to previous maladaptive behaviors. The psychosocial issues can also affect activities of daily living (ADL) performance. Learned ADL skills should be encouraged once the patient is home. Participation in activities outside of the home should be planned. The challenges of home life include the risk of isolation. Therefore, new routines formed in the psychiatric clinic or hospital should be continued once home.

Performing Activity Analysis in Relation to Occupation

Activity Analysis

An activity analysis is most commonly used in the return to work context or work hardening context. Although it can be used to determine if a client has the necessary performance components to perform any activity of daily living (ADL) or instrumental activity of daily living (IADL). The parts of an activity analysis may be broken down into three sections. First, it is important to determine the parts of an activity. For instance, does an activity require detailed memory recall, fine motor skills, heavy lifting, or exposure to dangerous chemicals? The next step is to determine if the client has the performance components necessary to complete the task. For instance, if a client has lower back pain, it is not realistic to expect them to return to a job lifting heavy boxes. Finally, the value of the activity must be assessed. If the activity is part of the client's employment, accommodations or compensatory methods may need to be explored.

Task Analysis for a Home Health Kitchen Evaluation

When evaluating the kitchen, safety is a primary concern. In addition to the physical components, the client needs to have the cognitive abilities to maintain safety during the entire task. A safety check for a smoke detector and fire extinguisher are the first steps in a kitchen assessment. It is important to evaluate kitchen space and whether the client can safely ambulate in a free, unobstructed area. Additionally, cookware and dishes should be located in a space that is easily reachable by the client. Cognition can be tested by having the client explain the steps to the chosen cooking activity. Organization, sequencing, memory, and attention are all important components of putting together a meal. As well, safety using sharp utensils and hot appliances should be examined. In the end, adaptive equipment such as built-up utensils, rocker knives, and large-handled appliance knobs may need to be recommended to compensate for physical deficits.

Task Analysis for Showering in a Shower Stall

The activity of showering in a shower stall involves the component of standing balance, transfer skills to the shower, active range of motion (AROM) with the user equipment (UE) to reach all parts of the body, sequencing skills to complete the correct order of the tasks, and cognitive skills for safety awareness during transfers as well as during the showering process. When standing balance

Copyright © Mometrix Media. You have been licensed one copy of this document for personal use only. Any other reproduction or redistribution is strictly prohibited. All rights reserved.
This content is provided for test preparation purposes only and does not imply an endorsement by Mometrix of any particular political, scientific, or religious point of view.

becomes impaired, it is often wise to recommend a shower chair to perform the showering task while seated. Grab bars are often added to the walls of the shower to safely transfer to and from the wet surface in the shower. Finally, it is important to make sure that the transfer surface outside of the shower is dry (before and after) the shower. Often, the floor outside of the shower can be kept dry with a non-skid mat. A non-skid mat also does not allow wet feet to slip on a slick floor.

Client Centered Collaboration

Continuity of Care in the Team Process

When team members work in their own specialty without collaboration, there is often duplication of services. This redundancy is frequently denied payment by insurance companies. Care that is well coordinated, however, is not duplicated or redundant but augments the efforts of other disciplines. This can only occur through communication and team meetings. For instance, a client receiving home health occupational therapy (OT) or physical therapy (PT) may be ambulating, as part of treatment, during each treatment. However, each discipline uses that treatment for a slightly different purpose. PT may use gait training to reduce the risk of falls by increasing balance. OT may use mobility training to negotiate obstacles in the kitchen. Both disciplines are using functional mobility for treatment but for a slightly different purpose. This level of collaboration occurs only through the communication/team process.

Multidisciplinary Model

The multidisciplinary team usually involves more than just the physician and occupational therapist (OT). In this type of model, there may be several team members (social worker, physician, OT, physical therapist, speech therapist, nurse, dietitian, and psychologist). The members of the team usually work separately to accomplish discipline-specific goals. In this scenario, all teamwork is done with the patient at the center of the model. However, communication among disciplines is minimal. This model is also not looked at as being effective. Therefore, the multidisciplinary model is not often used in a rehabilitation setting. This model is used in acute care settings in which more than one discipline of therapy may be ordered to treat a client. Care is directed by the physician and/or social worker. Collaboration on patient care may occur only one time a week—during a team conference.

Multidisciplinary Process

The multidisciplinary team approach is more collaborative. Team members work together to set goals and treatment as well as problem solve issues that may arise. The patient is at the center of the decision process. The patient's goals for treatment are kept in mind by all disciplines to allow the client to return to tasks that are important to them. All team members (including the physician) have equal roles on the interdisciplinary team. This model is most effective in a rehabilitation setting as it allows for a holistic approach that is patient focused. Team meetings to discuss the client occur frequently. The roles of each discipline are not in solo but in concert with each other. For instance, the occupational therapist may discuss methods for assisting a client to relearn how to make basic meals to return home alone after surgery. The physical therapist may work with the same client on mobility so that he or she does not fall when performing functional tasks. The social worker may work with the client on signing up for meals on wheels so that some of the stress of meal preparation is abated when first coming home from the hospital.

Medical Model

The medical model is a model in which communication is more vertical. The physician directs the care of the client and is at the center of all decisions. Although this model can be effective in a

Copyright © Mometrix Media. You have been licensed one copy of this document for personal use only. Any other reproduction or redistribution is strictly prohibited. All rights reserved.
This content is provided for test preparation purposes only and does not imply an endorsement by Mometrix of any particular political, scientific, or religious point of view.

setting in which the occupational therapist is part of a physician office, it is not effective in a setting in which multiple disciplines are involved. In a hospital or rehab setting, it is important for communication to be equal among all disciplines. The physician is one part of the team but not the most important team member. However, in a physician's office, there may be only one discipline (such as occupational therapy or physical therapy). The physician needs to write and direct all orders as well as oversee communication with family members. The patient is important but not at the center of the decision process.

Collaborative Process Between Teacher and OT in School Setting

The teacher is frequently met with the challenge of teaching a child with special needs. Deficits in areas such as writing, attention, self-control, toileting (and dressing associated with the task of toileting), and gross motor tasks associated with play and physical education all can be assessed and treated by the occupational therapist (OT). The teacher and OT frequently confer to determine the student's progress with acquiring and perfecting the skills necessary to be a good student. The OT acts more like a consultant in this environment. Treatments may occur one to two times per week. Treatment duration is determined only after close communication with teachers. The OT is free to recommend the involvement of other disciplines, such as speech or physical therapy.

Communicating Treatment Progress with OTR

The certified occupational therapy assistant (COTA) is responsible for communicating a client's progress toward goals as well as response to treatment to the occupational therapist, registered (OTR). The OTR is also responsible for arranging the required supervision of a COTA. Each state has slightly different requirements. However, the method for communication is generally the same. A COTA and OTR can communicate through written progress notes, verbal communication, and observation. Written communication is preferred as it can be documented in the patient chart. Written communication also allows for less discrepancy in interpretation of communication. Although each state may have a minimum requirement, it is better to communicate on a regular, frequent basis. The OTR also needs to observe to verify that treatments are delivered in the intended fashion to meet the client's goals and needs. There is no such thing as over-communication.

Communicating with Other Disciplines Involved in Client's Care

The first line of communication is always through the team conference. This is where members from all disciplines who are taking care of a client are able to gather and spend the time to discuss goals, problems, plan or treatment, and anticipated discharge of a client. Between team conferences, team members are encouraged to communicate through telephone, email, and text. It is important to keep in mind Health Insurance Portability and Accountability Act (HIPAA) standards when texting and emailing. Many times, encrypting messages that include patient names is best when using email as encryption increases security compliance. A good example of this occurs when the occupational therapist enters a patient's room and notices a change in medical condition of the patient. The nurse is consulted as well as the physician to determine what new changes in treatment are warranted. Care is maintained during all communication to make sure private information is not discussed in front of other clients.

Team Conference for Teenage OCD Client Returning Home after Short Stay in Psychiatric Unit

The team conference is a good place for family members to hear a summation of what was accomplished in therapy. Another goal of team conference is to review recommendations for further therapy. Team conference is also a great way for family members to voice concerns regarding the client's discharge from the hospital. Any 1:1 family training can also take place at this

Copyright © Mometrix Media. You have been licensed one copy of this document for personal use only. Any other reproduction or redistribution is strictly prohibited. All rights reserved.
This content is provided for test preparation purposes only and does not imply an endorsement by Mometrix of any particular political, scientific, or religious point of view.

time. Family training is not merely observing the therapist but is a time to perform hands-on assistance with issues such as transfers, instruction the client to better perform activities of daily living (ADLs) and instrumental activities of daily living (IADLs). Team conferences also involve the physician as well as social work services. Occupational therapists often assist social workers to set up a discharge that involves safe conditions for the client. A good example of this would be providing supervision for a client who has recently had a traumatic brain injury.

Scope of Practice

A scope of practice describes what a health care professional is permitted to do in keeping with the terms of his or her professional license. The scope of practice dictates what is legal and ethical for occupational therapists (OTs) to do in their everyday course of practice. With a scope of practice, limitations are set so that the profession is able to maintain a defined role for practitioners. This role is very different from that of other health care professions in that training has occurred within certain boundaries. For instance, an OT is not educated in gait training. Therefore, the expectation is that the physical therapist, who is trained in gait training, will train the patient in gait. With this in mind, it is clear that gait training is outside of the scope of an OT. State licensure boards oversee the adherence to the scope of practice and are responsible for administering fines for serious infractions.

Interdisciplinary Team Process for Prioritizing Goals for Clients

The interdisciplinary team always has to remain client centered. Information is gathered from the family, caregivers, and client to determine reasonable goals. Goals are determined by what is important to the client as well as what is feasible to accomplish in the time frame the patient will be in therapy. In the case in which there are multiple important goals, priority should be given to the more basic activities of daily living (ADL) goals. Although occupational therapists are trained to work on multiple goals simultaneously, basic ADLs need addressing prior to advanced tasks. With less time constraints, it may be possible to work on several ADL and instrumental activities of daily living (IADL) goals simultaneously (given safety is not a factor). This being stated, goals evolve and change depending upon progress and problems that arise during the rehabilitation process.

Ongoing Nature of the Collaborative Process

During the course of therapy, the interdisciplinary team can expect the client to make changes in physical, cognitive, and psychosocial abilities. The goals are for improvement of functional status. However, there are occasions in which there continues to be a decline (usually do to an ongoing illness) in abilities. The team should meet on a regular basis to determine short-term goals and modify existing goals according to the client's status. Although there is no set frequency that the team should meet, most interdisciplinary teams choose to meet on a weekly basis. Any frequency less than this would mean missing the opportunity to capitalize on possible gains. Mini (or informal meetings) may need to occur during the week to handle small issues that may arise between the more formal weekly meetings.

IEP and Role of OT

The role of occupational therapists (OTs) in the school is mainly supportive. As with most OT settings, the occupational therapist is part of the team comprised of the educators, parents, student, paraeducators, therapy staff, and administration. The Individualized Education Program (IEP) is required to meet periodically to discuss the student's plan for learning and the need for ancillary services (such as OT). The IEP meeting is the perfect place for the OT to discuss progress made toward therapy goals. It is also important to discuss integration of OT-acquired skills into the classroom. Any adaptations needed can be brought forth in from of the IEP members. This is a good place to modify or form new OT goals as the teacher may express deficit areas that an occupational

Copyright © Mometrix Media. You have been licensed one copy of this document for personal use only. Any other reproduction or redistribution is strictly prohibited. All rights reserved.
This content is provided for test preparation purposes only and does not imply an endorsement by Mometrix of any particular political, scientific, or religious point of view.

therapist can assist the student overcome. The goal is to assist the student to function to optimal levels to foster learning in the classroom.

Role of OT in Acute Care Discharge Planning

The occupational therapist (OT) plays a critical part in discharge planning from acute care settings. There are several key areas of concern. First, the OT recommends environmental changes as well as prescribes adaptive equipment. The OT is also concerned with transferring skills learned in the hospital setting to the home setting. One-on-one education is performed with family members to ensure the continuity of supervised and assisted skills. These skills may vary from activities of daily living (ADLs) to instrumental activities of daily living (IADLs) to transfers. Safety in areas of the home such as the bathroom and kitchen are important as the client may have a lack in judgment and safety due to recent illness or injury. Finally, the OT may assist team members in identifying family support issues as the burden of care of the client is transferred from the hospital to the client's family.

Discharge of Patient Prior to Meeting an OT Goal

With managed care shortening inpatient rehab days, it is important to prioritize occupational therapy (OT) rehab goals. However, there are occasions in which the patient is discharged home prior to meeting all goals. In these occasions it is important for the physician to order home health to continue therapy and continue reaching goals. A home program can be administered prior to discharge to help transition from inpatient rehab to home health. It is important to communicate any instructions for activities of daily living (ADLs) and instrumental activities of daily living (ADLs) to the client's caregivers. There may be several days or weeks before home health is initiated. The client's caregivers need to be prepared to perform the home program on a consistent basis not to lose any progress toward goals. A post discharge phone call from the therapist is useful for caregiver and client support.

Home Program for Cardiac Rehab Patient Graduating from Outpatient Program

The primary concern of a cardiac rehab program is to build aerobic capacity. Increasing endurance assists with stamina for everyday functional tasks. The heart is a muscle. When damaged by a myocardial infarction, it is important to strengthen undamaged tissues. Indoor and outdoor walking are good ways to maintain and build stamina. The parameters of exercise and cardiac response to exercise need to be taught to the patient. Signs and symptoms of over-exercise also need to be taught to equip the client with the knowledge necessary to stop the activity. Heart rate should be monitored on a regular interval during exercise. Target heart rate should be a percentage (determined by physician) of maximal heart rate. Knowledge of how to progress the walking program is the final step in the education process of a home program.

Responding to Patient Who is Not Comfortable Living at Home Without Assistance

There are many reasons a patient may feel uncomfortable being discharged from therapy. However, to understand the issues, it is important to listen to the reasoning given by the patient. Often other team members will need to assist in resolving the situation. For instance, if the issue centers on being home alone, a social worker may need to get involved to determine the availability and funds for home health or sitter services. If the issue is feeling lonely at home, then a psychologist may be useful to determine coping strategies. Finally, if the issue concerns safety in the home, a home evaluation can determine if further licensed services are warranted and under what type of setting (e.g., home health vs. outpatient). Remember, for therapy to continue, there must be functional goals unmet.

Copyright © Mometrix Media. You have been licensed one copy of this document for personal use only. Any other reproduction or redistribution is strictly prohibited. All rights reserved.
This content is provided for test preparation purposes only and does not imply an endorsement by Mometrix of any particular political, scientific, or religious point of view.

Responsibilities When a Client Wishes to Discontinue Occupational Therapy

The first responsibility you have as a certified occupational therapy assistant is to the well-being of the client. Although it is ultimately up to the client to decide whether or not they wish to continue occupational therapy services, a discussion of where he or she is in the attainment of long-term goals will need to be addressed. In some cases, the client may be close to meeting long-term goals. However, in other cases, there still may be goals to meet. This discussion should be introduced to the client as a first step. If the request to discontinue services is born out of frustration, goals may need to be modified to make them attainable. The occupational therapist, registered (OTR), will need to be involved and may need to discuss modification of goals with the client. The OTR will ultimately have to discharge the client if it is his or her wish.

Frequency and Duration for Home Health OT

The occupational therapist most typically will want to start therapy at a frequency and duration of three times a week for a few weeks. Although the home health certification period is 8 weeks, managed care dictates that there be a transitional decrease of treatment and frequency prior discharge. The length of therapy should not exceed the number of weeks absolutely needed to achieve goals. As goals are met, discharge should be planned. A 1-week notice is usually required by most insurance companies. The frequency of therapy should taper from three times a week to two times a week and then once a week to transition to a home program and/or outpatient therapy. In many cases, managed care dictates the total number of therapy sessions should not exceed a specific number of sessions (for occupational /physical /speech therapy combined). Therefore, close coordination of sessions among other team members is essential.

Strategies to Integrate Client into Therapy Program

The goals for a client are often ambitious (especially given the short stays of most hospital patients). It is important to judge a proper pace of therapy for the patient. Many patients will integrate well into the rehab environment. However, there will be the occasional client who states rehab is too tiring or too difficult. Pushing these patients to attend several therapy sessions in a row may only lead to patient refusals to attend therapy as well as over-fatigue. Instead, a slower-paced start to therapy is often better. At first, short sessions may lead to increased compliance. With time, lengthening sessions may provide for increased overall stamina for therapy. This is also part of the process of the client developing trust and rapport with the therapy team.

Prioritization of Goals

The goals of therapy are stated in relation to short- and long-term goals. Within the short-term goals, there may be some goals that need to be attained prior to others. For instance, for a stroke patient, the attainment of basic bilateral movement will precede controlled unilateral movement. For example, the patient will not be able to lift an affected arm to don a shirt without first attaining active range of motion (AROM) to the affected arm. A logical progression of treatment for goals should be discussed with the occupational therapist, registered and other team members to provide the best quality and continuity of care to the client. Patient input is also important as he or she may have a different priority of goals. In this situation, an agreement has to be reached with the client on the order of goal attainment.

Home Program for Client with Cognitive Impairments

A home program for a client with cognitive impairment will need to involve the caregivers. Because many cognitively impaired individuals require instruction over short periods of time, it is important to prepare the home program so that it can be divided into sections and implemented throughout the course of the day. Instructions should be simple one- or two-step commands. It is also

Copyright © Mometrix Media. You have been licensed one copy of this document for personal use only. Any other reproduction or redistribution is strictly prohibited. All rights reserved.
This content is provided for test preparation purposes only and does not imply an endorsement by Mometrix of any particular political, scientific, or religious point of view.

important to allow for gradations of the program upward as well as downward. Although the client will need to be able to follow instructions given for the home program, it will ultimately be up to the caregivers to understand all parts of the home program to instruct and implement the plan. Future appointments to adjust the home program may be necessary as improvements in cognition and/or activity level increase.

Monitoring Interventions

Effects of Time Constraints on Group Activities

A group activity should generally be completed within the time span of one treatment session. Some group projects may span two or more sessions. When planning on a group activity for one treatment session, consider that the introduction (or ice breaker), explanation of activity, actual activity, and post-activity discussion all need to occur within the time span of the 50 or so minutes allowed for the group. All preparation for a group should be made prior to the start of the group to avoid wasting the time of group members and to complete the requirements of the group within the allotted time frame. Finally, thought needs to be given to how much time needs to be given to each part of the group activity. Most of the time should be reserved for the actual activity.

Changing a Treatment Session to Hold the Client's Interest

Treatment plans involve a small degree of speculation about what will hold the interest and be a successful treatment of an individual. The more thorough the evaluation, the less the chance there is for planning a treatment session that is not successful. However, experienced therapists will always have a backup or second activity that they can fall back on if the primary planned treatment does not work. In fact, many times a review of previous skills learned not only enforces motor learning but also can serve as a good backup activity. Just like group activities, individual activities can span over the course of two or more sessions. A continuous activity that takes longer than one treatment session can begin to be monotonous. It is therefore recommended to perform more than one planned activity in a treatment session.

Process When Client is Unable to Participate in Prescribed Treatment

There may be some days that the client comes to therapy and feels ill or has had a regression and cannot fully participate in treatment. In this case, the certified occupational therapy assistant (COTA) needs to check with the occupational therapist, registered (OTR) to determine the best course of treatment. Any treatment that deviates from the plan should be discussed first with the OTR prior to implementation. That being said, many OTRs will write the treatment plan to cover a broad range of activities. This would account for the days that the client feels ill and needs to have an alteration to the normal course of treatment. The COTA, in conferring with the OTR, may assist the OTR to write new goals that account for the client's current change in condition. However, goals may not need to be revised if the client's change in condition is a temporary event.

Documentation of Progress in Group Activity

As in individual therapy, group therapy needs to be documented for each client. The standards for group therapy state that each client must have documentation related to the attainment of short- and long-term goals. Thus, the patient's role in a group setting should incorporate his or her goals. For instance, if a patient is working on attaining functional mobility in the kitchen, then the occupational therapist needs to have the patient stand and retrieve objects during a cooking group. The documentation for this patient would address activity performed in relation to goal attainment. If goals need to be revised, the occupational therapist, registered will have to provide input. Clear, concise documentation on the part of the certified occupational therapy assistant will make goal

Copyright © Mometrix Media. You have been licensed one copy of this document for personal use only. Any other reproduction or redistribution is strictly prohibited. All rights reserved.
This content is provided for test preparation purposes only and does not imply an endorsement by Mometrix of any particular political, scientific, or religious point of view.

revision easier. Groups can also have their own sets of goals that are documented each time the group meets. These goals should center on integrating the client back into the home environment as well as social situations.

Modifying Short- and Long-Term Goals of a Work-Hardening Patient

The main purpose of a work-hardening program is to return the client to work. More often than not, pain will be an issue in reaching goals. Assuming the client is not malingering, pain may be the reason for modifying short- and long-term goals. In situations in which there has been surgery or pain persists beyond the first few weeks of therapy, modification to the client's work environment may need to be considered. Adaptations to the workplace and/or adaptive equipment may be necessary on a temporary or permanent basis. In other cases, progress toward goals may take longer than planned and may require the alteration of the timeline to attain these goals. However, adaptive equipment and/or workplace modifications may still need to be made depending upon when the patient will require discharge from the program.

Monitoring Cardiac Patients for Attainment of Endurance-Related Goals

Occupational therapy assists cardiac patients to attain goals by analyzing activities, teaching energy conservation, teaching pacing, improving endurance for functional tasks, and teaching self-monitoring of vital signs for determining fatigue and when to rest. The attainment of these goals is the best way to monitor the achievement of increasing overall endurance. Pacing activities during the rehab process serves to allow quicker recovery as the heart has a chance to rest prior to over fatigue. The client should be taught to check his or her own pulse and blood pressure in response to activity. As cardiac fitness is attained, lower heart rates with activity will occur. As a result of increased cardiac fitness, the client will be able to increase activities with fewer rest breaks. This process should occur on a gradual and deliberate time frame.

Applying Adaptations to Lifestyle Changes

There are many times that we, as therapists, must be able to teach the client to adapt to lifestyle changes in response to disease progression. The goal of adaptation is to suggest a method for completing a task that is the least intrusive to a client's ability to perform a task. For instance, a client with diabetes may be taught how to prepare meals using a diabetic diet. Changes are not always drastic and should be the least invasive method possible. Research has shown that patients' compliance is often related to their perceptions of themselves and the amount of adaptation required. New, adaptive methods of performing leisure tasks is not always well received if the client is not able to derive the same enjoyment as previously. In these cases, learning new, less complex leisure skills is often the best substitute.

Behavioral Goals and Modifications for Left Hemiplegic Patients

Patients who suffer a stroke often have a change in personality. These clients can be emotionally labile, have short attention span, lack motivation, and easily feel frustrated. It is important for the occupational therapist to engage the client in activities that are stimulating but not overstimulating. Adjustments to mood, lability, and motivation will be gradual. Activities that encourage early success should be used to initiate rapport as well as confidence. Attention span is best improved through a combination of both neurocognitive therapy and occupational therapy together. Attainment of goals may be slower than planned and may require modification as well as an increased time period to achieve. If the patient experiences success, it is likely that he or she will also increase motivation as these two components are interrelated. Once motivation is achieved, goal attainment may be quicker.

Copyright © Mometrix Media. You have been licensed one copy of this document for personal use only. Any other reproduction or redistribution is strictly prohibited. All rights reserved.
This content is provided for test preparation purposes only and does not imply an endorsement by Mometrix of any particular political, scientific, or religious point of view.

Changes Over the Years in Therapy Needs for Children with Cerebral Palsy

As a child progresses from first grade through high school, he or she will physically develop and need additional splint or orthotic needs. This may include braces and/or wheeled mobility. Adaptations for play then turn to adaptations for school and the classroom. With advancing age, home programs that were once administered by caregivers can be learned by the patient. With age also comes the concern for appearance. Therefore, any braces, orthotics, and wheeled mobility will need to be designed with those qualities in mind. Also, with age, the client may be more willing to engage in increasingly intensive therapy. The teenage years may be a period of time for intensive therapy as tolerance and understanding for rehab increases.

Resources for Locating Precautions and Contraindications

Precautions and contraindications can be found in several resources. When available, it is always best to use the referring doctor's protocols. However, some physicians do not have specific protocols and rely on the therapist's knowledge. The easiest method for finding precautions is to look on the Internet. You do have to be careful of which source you use. Some sources are more reliable than others. If you stick with the big-name clinics and government agencies, you have a higher chance of accuracy. Sources such as Medlineplus.gov, Hopkinsmedicine.org, and healthfinder.gov are good general websites. Other sources are professional publications, professional organizations, and disease-specific websites. Most health care facilities also have small libraries specific to their clientele. Finally, online and live seminars offer great options for more detailed information concerning disease processes, precautions, and treatments.

Influences of Stages of Recovery on Precautions or Contraindications

The occupational therapist (OT) must be well versed on the clinic's protocols for precautions and contraindications associated with common diagnoses. Each doctor referring to the clinic has his or her own protocols. Some protocols may be totally different from one doctor to another. For instance, one surgeon may require early mobilization after a shoulder replacement, and another surgeon may require immobilization. There could even be variances with the same procedure and doctor. For instance, one client may have a partially torn ligament that is allowed to mobilize after 2 to 3 weeks post operation. Another client, using the same doctor, may have a completely torn ligament and is immobilized for 6 weeks. These nuances are important for the OT to know in daily practice. If there are any questions, it is better for the OT to contact the doctor than assume the answer.

Sternal Precautions After Cardiac Bypass Surgery

Sternal precautions help avoid excessive pressure that can separate the breast bone after open heart surgery. Actions to avoid are lifting more than five pounds, pushing or pulling, reaching behind the back or reaching with both arms out to the side, and reaching overhead. To maintain sternal precautions, the occupational therapist (OT) may assist with learning to roll in bed, transfer on and off the bed and toilet, and performing activities of daily living (ADLs) without breaking the precautions. The surgeon will further guide the patient as to specific precautions as well as length of maintaining sternal precautions. The home health OT can assist to make recommendations based upon the client's home environment. Adaptations in the form of raised surfaces (commode, chairs, and couches) may be necessary. Chair risers, a bedside commode, and proper transfer techniques are examples of interventions commonly recommended.

Copyright © Mometrix Media. You have been licensed one copy of this document for personal use only. Any other reproduction or redistribution is strictly prohibited. All rights reserved.
This content is provided for test preparation purposes only and does not imply an endorsement by Mometrix of any particular political, scientific, or religious point of view.

Selecting and Implementing Interventions

Promoting Healing and Enhancing Engagement

Selecting Appropriate Intervention Strategies

When determining intervention strategies, considerations such as diagnosis, theoretical model, and precautions are just the beginning. Based upon the current performance level, attention should be given to client preferences, age-appropriate interventions, and role-appropriate interventions. When several performance problems exist, priority must give to those issues requiring safety and independence that can be achieved within the time span the patient will be attending therapy. Although some issues need to be addressed while attending inpatient therapies, other goals can be attained on an outpatient or home health basis. Interventions that allow the patient to tap into available resources is also important. Rote exercise must be balanced with functional activities. Finally, previous therapist experience with various treatment models and interventions will assist to narrow the possibilities for treatment.

Preparing and Adapting the Intervention Technique

The method used for the intervention depends entirely on the status of the client. The same diagnosis may appear differently in each client. The ability to perform an activity analysis successfully is directly correlated to the ability to adapt an activity or exercise to the needs of each client. A complete review of the chart as well as the occupational therapist's evaluation will reveal the clinical findings as well as the treatment plan to follow. The ability to adapt an activity also is important as the client improves (or declines). Grading an activity is the next step after the activity is planned. Due to day-to-day changes that sometimes occur in a client's rehabilitation, it is a good idea to write down (informally) how the activity can be graded specifically.

Levels of OT Intervention

The first level of occupational therapy (OT) intervention involves adjunctive methods. Adjunctive methods are exercises, facilitation and inhibition techniques, modalities, splints, and sensory techniques. The second stage of OT intervention is enabling activities. These may not be considered purposeful activities but are steps toward the performance of purposeful activity. These involve performance components, such as dressing, using adaptive equipment. The third stage actually involves purposeful activity such as activities of daily living (ADLs) and instrumental activities of daily living (IADLs); these are used to evaluate, restore, and maintain the ability to function in life roles. The final stage of OT intervention involves the ability to perform occupations in the actual living environment. Although this is the ultimate goal, not all clients are able to achieve this level of activity. The determination of whether or not a client will reach the fourth stage is usually identified during the third stage.

Biomechanical Frame of Reference

The Biomechanical Frame of Reference emphasizes therapeutic exercise to improve range of motion, strength, and endurance. These elements, in turn, lead to improved functional abilities. This frame of reference is often used with orthopedic injuries such as rotator cuff tears, humeral repairs, shoulder replacements, and elbow and hand injuries or repairs. Although functional activities are incorporated into the treatment plan, rote exercise is also a substantial part of the treatment plan. The goals of treatments based upon this theory are to prevent limitation in range of motion, increase range of motion of a specific joint (or joints), increase strength, and increase endurance. Standard assessment tools include pain scales, manual muscle testing, and sensory testing. For

Copyright © Mometrix Media. You have been licensed one copy of this document for personal use only. Any other reproduction or redistribution is strictly prohibited. All rights reserved.
This content is provided for test preparation purposes only and does not imply an endorsement by Mometrix of any particular political, scientific, or religious point of view.

instance, a carpal tunnel surgery patient will often be taught nerve gliding exercises, active assistive range of motion, and scar massage.

Occupational Adaptation

Many events and conditions, such as illness or trauma, can impair the ability to adapt to role changes. Traditional models focus on improving skills such as sensorimotor, cognitive, and psychosocial systems. The Occupational Adaptation process directs treatment at affecting the internal ability to generate, evaluate, and integrate adaptive responses in which mastery of the environment is demonstrated. The occupational therapy focuses on the inner mechanisms that lead to the adaptation response by the patient. A successful adaptation response will eventually lead to mastery of the new situation. Because this process teaches the client to adapt, future challenges are better met with success. Functional performance is the main focus on therapy. For instance, a new stroke client may work on the functional task of making a bed to improve the areas of balance, gross motor, fine motor, sequencing, and functional mobility.

MOHO

The Model of Human Occupation (MOHO) was created by Dr. Gary Kielhofner in 1980. In this theory, humans are conceptualized as being made of the three components of volition, habituation, and performance capacity. Volition is the motivation for occupation. Habituation is the process in which occupation is organized into routines. Performance capacity refers to the physical and mental abilities that underlie occupational performance. This theory is designed for those people experiencing difficulty with their occupational lives. This theory can be applied to physical and psychological difficulties. The physical and social environments are emphasized in context to the occupations routinely performed to create a balance among volition, habituation, and performance capacity. This theory can be applied to all settings from the hospital and in-patient rehab to home health. There is also an associated screening tool that evaluates participation, performance, and skills associated with activities of daily living (ADLs) and instrumental activities of daily living (IADLs).

Treatment for Patient with Neck and Upper Back Pain from Sitting in a Chair and Typing

A thorough evaluation should include an evaluation of posture. Have the patient sit at a desk with a chair and computer placed in a similar position to the work space (or observe the patient on the job). Make note of postural issues due to improper alignment of equipment versus improper posture of the upper body. Strengthening exercises for the torso as well as the upper body will be important in conjunction with postural exercises. It will also be helpful to evaluate the patient typing to see if there are any overuse syndromes present from the combination of typing, improper posture, and/or improper height of equipment. The issues concerning equipment height may have to be addressed with the employer. Accessories such as the Varidesk allow for changing the height of the desk to allow working from a sitting as well as standing position.

Treatment Plan for Frozen Shoulder

The etiology of frozen shoulder is often unknown. However, it is important to know what stage of frozen shoulder the client exhibits. The first stage involves pain and inflammation with some decrease in motion. The second stage involves significant loss of range of motion with painful movements. This is the frozen stage. The last stage is thawing or regaining of motion. The goals of therapy are to decrease pain and inflammation; enhance blood flow to the shoulder through heat, massage, and light exercise; and teach the client a home exercise program that is not too aggressive in exercise but encourages movement. There are also numerous shoulder wraps that help relieve pain and inflammation as well as promote blood flow to the shoulder. Communicate with the

Copyright © Mometrix Media. You have been licensed one copy of this document for personal use only. Any other reproduction or redistribution is strictly prohibited. All rights reserved.
This content is provided for test preparation purposes only and does not imply an endorsement by Mometrix of any particular political, scientific, or religious point of view.

ordering physician on a regular basis to collaborate treatment and get the proper medicinal support to aid in the healing process.

Ensuring Patient's Privacy When Working Bedside

Hospital rooms area difficult places to ensure the privacy of a patient. Rooms are typically small, have many obstacles, and often are high-traffic areas. There are, however, a few rules to remember that help maintain a patient's privacy. First, most rooms have a curtain that can be drawn around the patient's bed. Although, the curtain can make a tight space even tighter, this is one way to ensure privacy. Another method is to take the patient into the bathroom and close the door. This option is not always feasible as the patient may not be able to get to the bathroom and require all therapy to be performed beside the bed. The last consideration would be to plan activities of daily living (ADL) activities at a time when the roommate will be out of the room (which is sometimes not possible)

Consideration for Male COTA Working with Female Client on Lower-Body Dressing

Activities of daily living (ADL) training with a client of the opposite sex can be challenging. Cultural values as well as beliefs help influence the client when it comes to ADL training. Some clients may be comfortable with a therapist from the opposite sex. Other therapists may wish to do training only with a therapist of the same sex. When clients feel modest, there are a few steps that can be taken to maintain privacy. First, if safety is not a concern, a curtain can be drawn during bathing or dressing certain parts of the body. Second, an aide who is of the same sex as the client may assist during parts of ADL training. Finally, some dressing training can be performed over existing clothing.

Wounds

Wounds provide their own set of challenges during the occupational therapy session. It is important to remember to wash your hands prior to treating a burn patient. Good hand hygiene is important to preventing infections. Do not manually stretch tissue that is not completely healed as this may cause a disruption in the healing process. Stretching is a prolonged process and requires splinting to maintain gains made in therapy. Manual stretching should be within the tolerance of the client but should be aggressive enough to prevent hypertrophic scarring. Some patients will tolerate deep heating tissues with ultrasound prior to stretching. Heat in the form of hot packs and steamed towels should be avoided over wounds as sensation may be compromised.

Stages of Burn Healing

Burn wounds are dynamic and change as they go through the stages of healing. The healing of first- and second-degree superficial burns is by primary intent. Second-degree superficial burns start the healing process from the epithelium of hair follicle remnants. Healing is complete in five to seven days. Second-degree deep burns as well as third-degree burns heal by secondary intent. This involves epithelization and contraction. All wounds go through the three stages of inflammation, proliferation, and maturation. Third-degree and some deep-tissue second-degree burns usually require skin grafts from healthy tissue to heal. Because tissues that heals over burn areas are not vascularized with blood vessels or innervated with nerve endings the same way as regular tissue, care must always be given to exposure to heat or cold.

Interventions for Superficial, Partial-Thickness Burns

Occupational therapists (OTs) play a significant role in burn care. The initial concern of burn care is to debride the wound bed by cleaning the remaining tissue and removing eschar (dead burned tissue). This allows for the growth of new tissue. Burns that are full thickness, as well as non-

Copyright © Mometrix Media. You have been licensed one copy of this document for personal use only. Any other reproduction or redistribution is strictly prohibited. All rights reserved.
This content is provided for test preparation purposes only and does not imply an endorsement by Mometrix of any particular political, scientific, or religious point of view.

healing partial-thickness burns, will often require skin grafts. The OT also assists with dressing changes. As part of therapy, gentle active and passive range of motion is important to all joints involved in the burns. This is helpful to prevent contractures. Splinting is also used when needed to prevent contractures and maintain a good alignment and stretch to involved tissues and joints. Finally, activities of daily living (ADLs) are incorporated into the therapy session to encourage the use of functional skills. Throughout treatment, it is very important to not only keep the wound clean but to keep it sterile to avoid secondary infection.

Facilitating ADLs into Treatment of Burn Patients

Activities of daily living (ADLs) are one of the best methods for follow-through of active motion and stretching. More gains in motion are achieved through functional movement and exercise combined than through exercise alone. The theory is that activity without purpose does not equate to anything more than raw exercise. For instance, the motion of forward flexion and abduction of the shoulder can be facilitated through donning and doffing a pullover shirt. Fine motor activity of the fingers can be facilitated through buttoning tasks. Upper extremity strengthening can be facilitated through donning and doffing pants. Assistance for each of these activities can be graded by the therapist depending upon the level of the patient. ADL activities also have a beneficial psychological effect for the burn patient as it brings forth capabilities the burn patient may have thought they permanently lost.

Hypertrophic Scar

A hypertrophic scar is one in which an overgrowth of tissue has occurred. A hypertrophic scar is thick and can limit range of motion. Deep, continuous pressure is one of the key treatments. This can be achieved through wearing compression garments. These garments are worn 24 hours a day for a few years. Active as well as passive range of motion is important to perform daily. Keeping the skin moist with lotion is also important during therapy as well as throughout the day. Surgical release of hypertrophic scaring is also an option if the scar has not stretched to the point of allowing full active range of motion.

Stages of a Pressure Ulcer

Pressure ulcers are classified in one of six stages. Stage one is intact skin with localized redness. The area of the wound is often more tender and is warm to the touch. Stage two is considered a partial-thickness burn. The tissue is shiny or dry but still shallow. Stage three involves the full thickness of the tissue as well as subcutaneous fat. The tendon, bone, and muscle may be exposed. Stage four is full thickness and often exposes underlying structures. This stage most often requires surgery. The next stage is "unstageable." This is due to the depth of the tissue being obscured by sloughing tissue or eschar. The final stage called suspected deep tissue injury. This stage is colored purple or maroon and often is accompanied by a blood blister. The full depth of the wound is gradually exposed as layers of skin blister and peel away.

Positioning Techniques to Avoid Decubitus Ulcers

Decubitus ulcers are most likely to occur in patients who stay in one place for a long time. Additionally, many of these patients have circulatory issues arising from diseases such as diabetes. Clients who are bed bound need to be turned every 1 to 2 hours. Those patients are who are wheelchair bound are usually taught how to perform pressure relief using their arms to push their buttocks up from the chair. Pressure relief needs to be performed for 30 seconds every 30 minutes. Patients who are bed bound with pressure sores need to be positioned so that they have no pressure on the wound. This is often accomplished by using bolsters and pressure-relieving boots. It is important to remember that the patient will likely be in a lot of pain and will need medication for pain relief prior to therapy.

Copyright © Mometrix Media. You have been licensed one copy of this document for personal use only. Any other reproduction or redistribution is strictly prohibited. All rights reserved.
This content is provided for test preparation purposes only and does not imply an endorsement by Mometrix of any particular political, scientific, or religious point of view.

Superficial Thermal Agents

Superficial heat modalities include hot packs, heating pads, paraffin bath, infrared and fluidotherapy. These modalities raise the body temperature and do not penetrate tissue more than 1 centimeter in depth. Heat is used for subcutaneous and chronic conditions and can reduce pain as well as relax tissues and joints. The most common cold modalities are cold packs, ice massage, cold baths, vapocoolant sprays, and cold compression units. These agents lower the body temperature. Applying hot or cold packs for 15 to 20 minutes is necessary to achieve the desired outcome. Ice massage usually occurs over a 7- to 10-minute time frame. Ice can be used to reduce acute inflammation and edema as well as reduce pain from muscle and ligament strain. Hot packs require the skin to be insulated from the packs themselves as the skin temperature tends to rise during the first few minutes of application as the heat penetrates the layers of insulation.

Contraindications for Use of Superficial Heat and Cold

Patients with peripheral vascular disease, bleeding disorder, malignancy over the site of heat, acute inflammation or trauma, edema, infection, open wounds, large scars or with impaired sensation (neuropathy) or impaired ability to communicate (dementia) should avoid superficial heat. These patients have the increased risk of burns from the heat. Contraindications for cryotherapy are poor tolerance to cold, Raynaud's disease, peripheral vascular disease, open wounds, impaired sensation, and impaired ability to communicate. The certified occupational therapy assistant (COTA) must always follow the treatment plan of the occupational therapist, registered (OTR). If the COTA feels a patient may benefit from a modality, it is important to discuss this suggestion with the OTR so that the treatment plan can be updated to include these modalities.

Use of Paraffin for Arthritis

A paraffin bath is useful in treating the symptoms of pain associated with forms of arthritis. The paraffin bath should be set for the temperature of 125 degrees Fahrenheit. Care must be given when the client first immerses a hand into the bath as the hand will need to adjust to the temperature of the wax. The hand is dipped about ten times into the wax and then covered with plastic wrap and a towel for insulation. Generally, heat will dissipate after 10 minutes. The wax can be used only once as replacing the wax into the bath is an infection control issue. There are times when the hand may be wrapped in a flexed position to facilitate wrist and/or finger flexion. This is usually accomplished with the use of an elastic sports wrap.

Fluidotherapy

Fluidotherapy uses a stream of heated air flowing over and through fine grains of a material called Cellex. This stream creates air pockets and bubbles to provide a comfortable massage. Range of motion is often performed during fluidotherapy. The machine for fluidotherapy can be set to different modes from pulse to vibrate. Fluidotherapy is a superficial heat and can be used to increase range of motion as well as decrease pain. The buoyancy of the limb in the fluidotherapy machine allows for range of motion exercises as well as hand strengthening as objects can be placed in the machine for exercise. Massage also increases circulation. It is important for the patient not to have any open wounds as this would lead to cross-contamination.

Working on Hand Active Range of Motion While Using Fluidotherapy

Fluidotherapy machines for the hand usually have a big enough space inside to place objects that can be manipulated and squeezed to work on hand motion and strengthening. Foam balls are a good way to work on non-resistive active range of motion. Soft rubber balls can be graded in density to not only work on active range of motion but also strengthening. Fluidotherapy also involves the blowing of heated air, which helps the corn husks to massage the entire hand as well as

Copyright © Mometrix Media. You have been licensed one copy of this document for personal use only. Any other reproduction or redistribution is strictly prohibited. All rights reserved.
This content is provided for test preparation purposes only and does not imply an endorsement by Mometrix of any particular political, scientific, or religious point of view.

relax the hand and allow scar tissues to stretch. Fluidotherapy is usually used as a precursor or warm-up activity and usually followed with therapist-led stretching and exercise. Fluidotherapy can be used safely for 15 to 20 minutes as long as the heat setting is monitored to ensure the temperature does not get too hot for the client.

Addressing Redness After Use of Hot Packs

Hot packs increase circulation and can cause temporary blanching or red areas of the skin. These areas should clear within about 10 minutes. If the redness does not go away, the clinical supervisor as well as the ordering physician should be notified. Prior to application of hot packs, it is important to note any red areas on the skin, lacerations, and contusions. This step is important to prevent future liability issues post-treatment. The treatment note also needs to include the time hot packs were on the patient as well as the skin condition post treatment. Finally, it is contraindicated to use hot packs in conjunction with transcutaneous electrical nerve stimulus (TENS), ultrasound, or any other heat modality. The combination of heat modalities used at the same time could cause superficial as well as deeper burns.

Use of Hot and Cold Packs for Post Shoulder Replacement Client with Orders for Active Assistive Range of Motion

Because hot packs are most often used to relax tissues, they would be most effective prior to any exercise. Tissues respond better to exercise as well as stretching if they are warmed first. Without taking the time to use hot packs, tissues remain stiff and have an increased risk of tearing when stretched. Cold packs are best used post treatment and are used to reduce inflammation and pain that occurs with exercise. Hot packs require the presence of a licensed therapist because there is the risk for burns due to the initial rising temperature of tissues covered by the packs. Also, be aware that a fresh surgical wound may be more sensitive to heat and require more insulation from the hot packs. Finally, it is important for the administering therapists to document the condition of the skin both pre- and post-administration of the hot packs.

Contrast Bath

Contrast baths are used to decrease pain, swelling, inflammation, and improve mobility. A contrast bath is set up with two tubs of water—one warm and one cold (ice cold). The injured part of the body is lowered into the warm water first. It should be left in the water for 3 to 4 minutes. Then, the patient moves to place the injured limb into the cold water. Typically, the limb is left for about 1 minute in the cold water. This sequence of warm to cold is done for about 30 minutes. After the bath, it is always important to follow through with functional activities and exercise. You should look to see if the contrast bath had the desired effect. Documentation should include water temperature as well as procedure. State any therapeutic gains made by the bath.

Infrared Therapy

Infrared therapy is the use of infrared light to treat chronic and acute pain and is a fairly new form of therapy. A 30-minute session increases circulation by 400 percent to the treated area. This allows for pain reduction as well as healing of tissues. Multiple treatment sessions are required to derive benefit. This treatment is effective for arthritis, back pain, bursitis, carpal tunnel, rheumatoid arthritis neck pain, tendinitis, surgical wounds, and so on. Because infrared light is a thermal treatment, care must be given to not overheat tissues. Because of the intensity of the light, be sure to not gaze directly into it as this can cause eye strain. This type of therapy can also be performed by the patient at home.

Copyright © Mometrix Media. You have been licensed one copy of this document for personal use only. Any other reproduction or redistribution is strictly prohibited. All rights reserved.
This content is provided for test preparation purposes only and does not imply an endorsement by Mometrix of any particular political, scientific, or religious point of view.

Deep Thermal Therapy

Deep heat agents are ultrasound and phonophoresis. Ultrasound is the use of sound waves to treat musculoskeletal pathology. Ultrasound serves the purpose of increasing circulation for wound healing as well as decreasing pain. A handheld transducer is moved in a circular motion over the injured area. The transducer produces sound waves that heat deep tissues. Contraindications for ultrasound are impaired sensation, cancer, pacemaker, metal implants over the affected site, and decreased cognition. Phonophoresis is the application of ultrasound to enhance the delivery of topical drugs. Dexamethasone (an anti-inflammatory drug) is often used to reduce inflammation. The drug is in a gel form and rubbed into the affected area. Ultrasound waves dilate blood vessels, which in turn, enhances the uptake of the drug. Contraindications are much the same as ultrasound with the added precaution of not getting the medication around the eyes or mouth.

Advantages and Disadvantages of CPM Machines

Continuous passive motion (CPM) machines are commonly used for shoulder replacements as well as joint replacements of the hand. CPMs perform mechanical motion to the operated joint. The range of shoulder flexion and extension is determined by the prescribing physician and may be adjusted as prescribed. The pace of the motion is usually slow but can be increased or decreased as necessary. Studies have shown the best compliance with therapy when the CPM machine is connected to the individual early after surgery. This is why, many times, clients wake up from surgery with these machines attached to the operated joint. CPMs are used several times a day for one to two hours at a time. Once active motion is allowed, time on the CPM machine is gradually tapered.

Fitting Procedure for Continuous Passive Range of Motion Machine for the Hand

The passive range of motion machines or continuous passive range of motion (CPMs) are designed to be placed in a specific manner on the hand, wrist, or fingers. Depending upon the necessity, the CPM is aligned with the joint in the same plane with the bones leading to and from the joint. Care is observed to make sure the alignment of the joint of the machine is over the joint of the body part that is being moved. The settings for flexion and extension must be within the tolerance and discretion of the therapist and patient. It is important to stretch the joint slightly but not overstretch as to break down healing tissues and cause scar tissue and pain. CPMs are worn for several hours during the course of a day for best results.

Qualifications to Use Physical Agent Modalities

Occupational therapists and assistants must demonstrate competence in using modalities prior to using them with patients. Education consisting of continuing education courses, classes at conferences, and accredited higher education courses or programs must be taken to qualify to use modalities. Education on each modality that consists of the biophysical, neurophysical, and electrophysical changes that occur as a result of using the modality must be documented for the occupational therapist to gain credit for this learning activity. Indications, contraindications, and precautions are essential to any course training in modalities. Finally, education on documentation—to include elements of documentation, parameters for intervention, subjective and objective criteria, efficacy, and the relationship between the modality and performance—must be included in any program for learning modalities.

Ultrasound Procedure

Ultrasound is performed with the use of a water-based gel that acts as a medium for passing the ultrasonic current into the area being treated. The area being treated is usually two times the size of

Copyright © Mometrix Media. You have been licensed one copy of this document for personal use only. Any other reproduction or redistribution is strictly prohibited. All rights reserved.
This content is provided for test preparation purposes only and does not imply an endorsement by Mometrix of any particular political, scientific, or religious point of view.

the head of the transducer with the treatment lasting around 8 to 10 minutes. The head is always moved in a slow motion. Care is given to not stop moving the transducer as this may lead to discomfort and burns. Documentation consists of describing the area of body being treated, frequency, intensity, duration, and patient response. If medication is used (phonophoresis), the medication name and dosage is described. Finally, ultrasound should be used only over the tissues of fascia, joint capsules, ligaments, scar tissue, and tendons. Never perform ultrasound over bone.

TENS

Transcutaneous electrical nerve stimulation (TENS) is the use of electrical current to stimulate nerves for therapeutic reasons. Most often TENS is used to break the pain cycle by interrupting the pain pathway with electrical pulses. At higher frequencies, this device stimulates nerve contraction and can be used in conjunction with neuro re-education. TENS for pain is used over a long period of time, whereas TENS for stimulation, a higher wattage, is used for a shorter period of time. There are several contraindications for TENS. TENS should not be used over the cranial area, with patients who have a pacemaker, or over lesions and should not be placed over the carotid sinus or over the anterior aspect of the neck. Additionally, clients with decreased sensation or cognitive impairments should not be treated with TENS before consulting their physicians.

Implementing Strategies to Support Participation in ADLs

Role of Leisure in Daily Routine

Leisure is an important part of a daily routine for people of all ages. As people develop infirmities, such as low vision, stroke, and orthopedic problems, it is often harder to perform the leisure activities as prior to the illness. Many times, adaptations can be made to perform the same activities. However, there are times where it may be difficult or unsafe to participate in the same leisure tasks. Occupational therapists play an important role in assessing skill levels and recommending adaptations or the participation in alternative leisure activities. For many seniors, leisure activities are the way they are connected to the world around them. Leisure activities often involve socialization and cognitive skills that keep the mind sharp. Studies have indicated that people with leisure interests have better coping skills as well as are happier than those with no leisure interests.

Helping Clients with Few Leisure Skills Develop Leisure Skills to Cope with Recent Illness

The first step the occupational therapist (OT) should do is to perform a skills or leisure inventory. Assessments such as the Leisure Skills Checklist, the OT Assessment Index, Skills and Experience Inventory, and the Kohlman Evaluation of Living Skills are useful to identify strengths and weaknesses with relation to skills used for leisure. These assessments can also be used to determine what strengths can be developed to participate in meaning leisure tasks. The objective nature of these inventories will often produce incite that has been previously unexplored and that can be of benefit to the client. Leisure skills do not always stay the same. Instead, they evolve over time and have a direct relation to situations that affect a client's physical and psychological well-being. As such, the OT facilitates self-exploration of skills to maximize abilities.

Grading

Grading means to increase or decrease the difficulty of an intervention depending upon how the patient responds to the task. If an activity is too easy, you will want to make it a greater challenge. If the activity is too hard, it may be difficult or unsafe to complete and require downgrading. An appropriate grade for an activity will have some challenge but not be too difficult to complete. For

Copyright © Mometrix Media. You have been licensed one copy of this document for personal use only. Any other reproduction or redistribution is strictly prohibited. All rights reserved.
This content is provided for test preparation purposes only and does not imply an endorsement by Mometrix of any particular political, scientific, or religious point of view.

instance, a patient who is given the task of standing to perform hygiene at a sink may not be able to stand the entire duration of the task. The task can be downgraded to allow for some sitting time when the patient gets tired. When the patient has better tolerance for the standing portion of the task, he or she may be progressed to standing for longer periods of time.

Medical Factors

A client's performance completing an activity or exercise can be affected by several medical factors. Weight-bearing status, fall precautions, and no food by mouth orders are some of the factors that can affect how an activity is graded. Other factors include pain, current adaptive equipment required to complete a task, the amount of assistance needed to complete the task, cognitive level, and any changes in medical condition. It is up to the certified occupational therapy assistant (COTA) treating the patient to determine how the client is doing, on any given day, and to make changes to the activity as needed. It is also important to realize that several factors may interplay and require further upgrading or downgrading of the activity. The COTA should also consult the occupational therapist, registered to make changes, as needed, to the treatment plan.

Grading Cross-Friction Massage on Client with Lateral Epicondylitis

Cross-friction massage is a technique used on sore muscles, tendons, and ligaments to support the healing of torn fibers. Lateral epicondylitis can be very painful. Pain as well as healing is often decreased with massage. Cross-friction massage is successful because the cross section of fibers is massaged, allowing for increased blood flow as well as pain reduction. There are times, however, where the massage can hurt because the therapist is using too much force. When this occurs, the activity can be graded to allow for a lighter massage. Keep in mind that a massage that hurts actually defeats the purpose of the massage by causing more irritation and discomfort. In turn, this can increase the amount of time required to heal.

Grading a Cooking Activity for 10-Year-Old Cerebral Palsy Patient

A 10-year-old cerebral palsy patient likes to assist her mother bake cookies. This patient is having increased difficulty walking and now performs most activities from a wheelchair level. This patient is a good example of someone who has the knowledge of how to perform a task but, due to a decline in functional status, is requiring the activity to be downgraded as her condition changes. Making cookies is an activity that can be adapted to a tabletop level. The mixing of ingredients can be performed from a sitting level. Placing items in the oven will need to be assessed for safety. However, assuming there are no safety concerns, the placing of the cookies in the oven can also happen from a wheelchair level. The cleanup after the activity may involve some standing but can also mostly be performed from a sitting level. Standing should be encouraged, as tolerated, with tasks that do not pose a safety risk while trying to maintain balance in this position.

Considerations for Diabetes Patients and Cooking Tasks

It is important to start with a good standing surface. Good shoes that offer support help provide stable standing support. A stool to sit on during the cooking activity may be necessary if standing fatigue is an issue. Sharp knives pose a risk for injury. It may be wise to purchase pre-cut foods. Be careful to avoid touching objects that are either too hot or too cold. It is important to remember that safety is most important as sensation to the hands is often reduced and the ability to feel hot objects may be impaired. A hand mitt may need to be worn to protect the hands from objects that are at temperature extremes. Many stores will also carry utensils for cooking that have built-up or enlarged handles.

Copyright © Mometrix Media. You have been licensed one copy of this document for personal use only. Any other reproduction or redistribution is strictly prohibited. All rights reserved.
This content is provided for test preparation purposes only and does not imply an endorsement by Mometrix of any particular political, scientific, or religious point of view.

Tactile Defensiveness

Children who are tactile defensive are hypersensitive to touch (tactile input). These children will often avoid that which involves textures: hugging, kissing, tags on clothing, socks, shoes, seams on clothing, play dough, sand, and hands or face being dirty. Exposure to these types of sensory input will evoke anxiety, fear, and avoidance. Tactile defensiveness limits the learning and sensory maturation process. Tactile defensiveness is treated with deep pressure, weighted objects, light brushing, and a slow introduction to sensory experiences. With slow, gradual grading of tactile activities, the child is better able to integrate textures into the routine of normal activities. For instance, a soft cotton ball can be used to start the tactile experience as it is very soft. As the child becomes used to this, toys such as play dough can eventually be integrated.

Group Therapy

There are several advantages to placing clients in a group therapy situation. First, the diversity of opinion allows for psychosocial-related groups to share ideas and thoughts with their group members. In all therapy groups (addressing psychosocial and/or physical dysfunction) there can be the building of camaraderie and support. This comes from the fact that group members will usually have similar diagnoses. It is the sharing of ideas that group members begin to feel connected. However, with experience, therapists learn to look for personalities of group members that may clash. When the group is interrupted with clashing personalities, it makes it very difficult to perform planned activities. This is a good reason to keep the group small (when possible). However, when there is the need for a larger group, additional therapists may need to be utilized to maintain the flow of the planned activity as well as assist with clients who may need closer supervision during the group activity.

Group Formats

The thematic group assists group members to acquire a specific skill. The group is designed to train in a specific skill that can transfer to outside of the group. The topical group is a discussion group that discusses an activity and solution to problems associated with engaging in the specific activity. Skills are also transferable to community activities. The task-oriented group increases the client's awareness of needs, values, ideas, feelings, and behavior as they engage in the task. Tasks simulate real-life scenarios. The developmental group teaches interactive skills to group members. A parallel group is one in which group members perform individual tasks in the presence of others but have minimal interaction with group members. Finally, the project group is designed to perform a shared group activity in a cooperative manner. Members of this group assist each other.

Group Setting Considerations

There are several key factors that need to be determined when arranging an occupational therapy group. First, it is important to define the purpose and target audience of a group. Second, it is equally important to define the age group the activity will be designed for. Defining the purpose, target audience, and age group allows the occupational therapist to tailor the group activity to the needs of group members. It is also important to define the time length for each group session. The activities selected must conform to the length of time allowed for each group. Finally, the group activity must have a method to grade upward or downward. It will be necessary during the course of several groups to grade the activity for the use of clients who need more of a challenge as well as to clients who need less of a challenge.

Age-Appropriate Group Activities

For a group activity to be meaningful, it must be appropriate to the age of clients who participate in the group. Groups can be designed for functional activities such as cooking, gardening, self-care,

Copyright © Mometrix Media. You have been licensed one copy of this document for personal use only. Any other reproduction or redistribution is strictly prohibited. All rights reserved.
This content is provided for test preparation purposes only and does not imply an endorsement by Mometrix of any particular political, scientific, or religious point of view.

functional mobility, and so on. Groups can also be designed for exercise such as chair-level strengthening exercises. However, it is important to make all material relevant to the age range of the group. For instance, you would not want to engage elderly men in a gardening group if they do not have an interest in such an activity. The attention group members devote to a group is directly related to the interest in that group. Furthermore, group activities should not be demeaning and insulting in any way. For instance, adults may not want to participate in a cognitive group designed for basic orientation (if cognitive levels are not an issue) but may enjoy an activity such as trivia.

Group Seating to Facilitate Communication for a Group of 10

The group setup will be decided based upon type and size of the group. If there are a large number of clients in a group that requires sharing of ideas, it may be best to divide the larger group into smaller, individualized subgroups. If space allows, a circular setup is also ideal to facilitate conversation. However, a group facilitator may be necessary to ensure all participants have a chance to contribute to the group. Additionally, as a rule, groups should be located in areas of the therapy center that will not disturb other therapists and patients. Finally, with a group of 10 patients, it would be best to have two facilitating therapists (or one therapist with an aid). The setup should be prearranged prior to the arrival of clients as this will save valuable time for the group activity. Be flexible and allow for last-minute changes based upon participants in the group.

Handling Clients Who are Not Participating and Reluctant to Perform Group Activities

This is a situation that all therapists will eventually experience. Planning and forethought can help make the transition in this situation smoother. No one enjoys feeling left out of a group. There usually is a reason for not participating in a group activity. For some, the activity may seem too challenging. These individuals may need the activity graded in such a way that they are able to participate with modifications. Other individuals may not understand the instructions and need further explanation. It also may be necessary to remove individuals from the group and provide the necessary guidance away from the group to not disturb the activity in progress. Sometimes, individuals turn out to be inappropriate for the group and need to be separated and provided another task to perform.

Advantages to Group Setting in Mental Health Occupational Therapy

Recent studies have indicated the brain has more of a capacity for change in a group activity. Individual activities are sometimes necessary in a mental health setting. However, as the brain is hardwired for social networking, learning can often take place more efficiently in this context. Empathy allows individuals to share stories and experiences that activate the frontal, temporal, and somatosensory cortex as well as the amygdala. Individuals can actually suppress their views and empathize with others. This focus away from an individual's own problems and onto finding solutions for others helps in the individual's learning process. Therefore, a hands-on method for learning takes place in a group environment. New neurons can actually be formed as group activities and discussions modify and form new behaviors.

Considerations for Group Activities in Psychiatric Setting

In a psychiatric setting, there are several considerations that need to be made prior to choosing a group activity. First, consider the age and sex of group members. This will help determine age-appropriate activates as well as activities appropriate for the male and female sex. Group activities should be centered on the topics of education, anger management, self-care, and cohesiveness. It is important to know how to diffuse triggers that may, inadvertently, break down communication among group members. Worksheets, relaxation exercises, yoga, expressive group activities, and games (i.e., charades) all are activities that lend themselves well to groups. Always have more than

Copyright © Mometrix Media. You have been licensed one copy of this document for personal use only. Any other reproduction or redistribution is strictly prohibited. All rights reserved.
This content is provided for test preparation purposes only and does not imply an endorsement by Mometrix of any particular political, scientific, or religious point of view.

one possible group activity ready to go as there will be times when what was planned does not work out. Instead a second or third choice activity is preferred.

Dividing Activities for a Group Cooking Activity

Suppose you are the occupational therapist in a rehab center and are planning a cooking activity with four clients for your morning session. Your group will have stroke patients. The first thing to do in this situation is to write down the tasks involved with the cooking activity. For instance, cooking eggs might involve the steps of retrieving materials, cracking and scrambling the eggs, cooking the eggs, and cleaning up. These five tasks can be divided among the four clients depending upon their abilities and therapeutic goals. A patient with a goal of walking may be in charge of retrieving materials, a patient with the goal of increasing upper body strength may be in charge of scrambling the eggs. The tasks assigned will be dependent also upon the current level of the patient as well as any safety concerns. It is generally a good idea to debrief patients after the group activity is completed by discussing the successes as well as areas for improvement.

Planning for Traumatic Brain Injury Group Working on Functional Mobility and Environmental Safety

The first thing to determine is the number of clients and the number of therapists that will be attending the group. There may be a need for some clients to have 1:1 attention during the group. Other clients may be able to be paired with another individual and a therapist between them. The next step is to determine goals. A person who is wheelchair bound may have a goal of safety during mobility, attending to a neglected side, and not running into objects with the wheelchair. A person with a goal of walking may have deficits in balance and may have a goal of using the walker to practice transfers to surfaces (including the bathroom and bedroom). This is the type of group that can be multidisciplinary by including both occupational therapist and physical therapist.

Visual Motor Skills

Visual motor skills help interpret forms, shapes, figures, and objects. Visual motor skills also include the coordination of visual information that is perceived and processed with motor skills that include fine motor, gross motor, and sensory motor tasks. Most physical activities involve the integration of visual motor skills. This is why play is so important. Play allows for exploration as well as the ability to practice visual motor skills. Visual motor skills also include eye-hand coordination development. Spatial relations is a term that has to do with the perception of the body in space. Figure ground is the ability to locate objects within clutter. Finally, visual closure involves the ability to fill in parts of a form when the whole shape is not given.

Intervention Activities for Improving Visual Motor Skills

For children, age-appropriate visual motor skills allow for the ability to engage in sports, complete puzzles, color within lines, and write legibly. Jumping games such as jumping jacks and jump rope help develop visual motor skills by challenging the balance (vestibular mechanism) of the brain. Hand-strengthening activities such as playing with play dough assist in developing hand strength that will eventually be used in writing. In general, catching activities develop eye-hand coordination to engage the child in sports at an early age. Large blocks are also a good way to begin to develop visual motor skills as well as allow for creativity in building structures. Slides and trampolines are good methods to develop spatial relations; this also helps develop the vestibular system.

Compensatory Techniques for Visual Field Loss

About 20% to 30% of patients undergoing rehabilitation after a brain injury experience a homonymous hemianopsia. This is characterized by loss of the same half of the visual field in both eyes. The rehabilitative phase focuses on optimizing the patient's function by techniques such as

Copyright © Mometrix Media. You have been licensed one copy of this document for personal use only. Any other reproduction or redistribution is strictly prohibited. All rights reserved.
This content is provided for test preparation purposes only and does not imply an endorsement by Mometrix of any particular political, scientific, or religious point of view.

focusing on the blind field of vision to allow for increased awareness of scanning all visual fields more evenly. Optical aids such as prisms also serve to extend quality of vision. In general, rehabilitation is aimed at compensatory techniques. Although recent research has shown that compensatory techniques may not prove as effective as once thought, it remains the primary mode of rehabilitation for visual field loss. Additionally, there remains a poor prognosis for patients with visual field loss. Few patients recover full visual field function.

Perceptual Processing

Perceptual processing is the subjective, active, and creative process through which individuals assign meaning to sensory information. The first stage is stimulation. This stage involves contact with a particular stimulus that can be from any sense. Stage two is organization. In this stage, the capacity to identify and recognize objects and events is important for normal perception. Perception errors can affect what individuals perceive from their senses. The next three stages are interpretation-evaluation, memory, and recall. These stages are related as the evaluation of stimuli depends upon previous memory as well as what can be recalled from previous situations. Perception influences all stages and accounts for the differences in interpretation among individuals. Other factors influencing perceptual processing are knowledge, culture, and beliefs.

Sensory Arousal

The brain organizes information that is processed from the environment. This information is obtained from senses. These senses bombard the brain at any given moment with many impulses. The ability for the brain to make sense of these impulses and the ability to act appropriately to stimuli is what is called sensory arousal. When the brain perceives too much disorganized information at one time, it can seem like a "traffic jam." When the brain is slow to perceive information, this is a lower state of arousal. This state often is associated with slower cognitive functioning. The brain has the ability to self-regulate sensory stimuli by shutting out unnecessary stimuli to focus on necessary sensations. The refinement of this process usually occurs at the age of eight.

Intervention Activities to Decrease Sensory Arousal

Overstimulation of the senses can be caused by the inability to process information at the organizational stage. With children who have this type of problem, information is perceived but not interpreted in an organized fashion. Therefore, the sensory system is overloaded. Therapy involves teaching family and caregivers to reduce stimuli and introduce new stimuli in a slow and organized fashion. The senses often need quiet, gentle sounds as well as soothing colors and smells to reprogram the brain to process information in an orderly fashion. These children are not always integrated into a regular classroom and sometimes need special education in an environment adapted for them. This type of environment usually has special, soothing lighting as well as reduced stimuli and a learning environment that is slower paced.

Intervention Methods to Increase Sensory Arousal

Intervention methods to increase sensory arousal include gentle rocking, deep pressure, swinging, rolling, and tumbling. These are some of the basic movements that are used to increase arousal. Items used in conjunction with these movements are balls, bolsters, tumbling bolsters, and swings hung from the ceiling. Movements are graded so that the senses are not overloaded. The movements need to be slow but deliberate. As the sensory system develops, larger, quicker movements are introduced into the therapy session. Oral motor skills are also necessary to develop with these children. The skills of sucking, chewing, and blowing are often delayed and need therapeutic intervention. In many cases, early intervention can lead to improved attention, motor skills, and improved play skills. Delays in learning skills also are minimized by early intervention.

Copyright © Mometrix Media. You have been licensed one copy of this document for personal use only. Any other reproduction or redistribution is strictly prohibited. All rights reserved.
This content is provided for test preparation purposes only and does not imply an endorsement by Mometrix of any particular political, scientific, or religious point of view.

Sensory Integration

Sensory integrative disorder is the inability for the brain to integrate information from the body's senses of sight, smell, sound, taste, temperature, position, and movements of the body in space. Movements such as rocking, kneeling, doing activities on the stomach, and performing activities on or with therapy balls have all been effective strategies that occupational and physical therapists have used to treat sensory integrative problems. A home program (sensory diet) will often be prescribed by the therapists that allows parents to perform a set of activities with their child aimed at increasing attention, arousal, and adaptive responses. Many children who have sensory integrative problems are on the autistic spectrum, have attention-deficit hyperactivity disorder (ADHD), and have learning disabilities. Sensory integration is important to work on in the early years of life as success in school depends on the skills acquired during early motor learning.

Sensory Integrative Issues Related to Touch

Touch is very important as it is one way individuals interact with the world. On a daily basis, the average person touches many items that are of many different consistencies. For those kids with sensory integrative problems, touching different textures is difficult. These kids often exhibit avoidance behaviors to touching textured items. Therapy for this issue involves playing with items such as play dough, clay, and sand. These items allow the child to use play to integrate progressively more challenging textures into the realm of touch. Avoidance to certain textures is addressed as the child is challenged to play with rougher textures as they progress and tolerate. The home program often involves play and is rewarded as the children challenge themselves and overcomes the sensitivity to textures.

Treating Childhood Feeding Problems

The signs that a child is having a feeding disorder are growth issues, abnormal sucking and swallowing, gagging during feeding, difficulty transitioning from pureed food to solid foods, and refusal to eat certain textured foods. An occupational therapist (OT) performs feeding therapy for 30 to 60 minutes one to two times per week. Exercises that strengthen the mouth musculature such as blowing bubbles, whistling, and making silly faces are sensory integrative in nature and good as a precursor to feeding skills. Foods of different textures are gradually introduced to the child. OTs play an important role in also educating the parents about home programs to promote feeding skills. Rewards serve to reinforce gains made in therapy and at home. The importance of positive reinforcement can make a difference between a child having a good or a bad experience with therapy.

Sensory Demands of a Birthday Party

Children with sensory integrative problems can easily be overwhelmed by the stimuli at a birthday party. New noises and large numbers of people can be overwhelming. Additionally, new foods such as cake and ice cream can pose a problem as sudden diet changes can affect the behavior of a child. Organized games are often not successful as they demand attention that just is not there (especially while in a stressful environment). Finally, the ability to allow the child to come and go at will enable the child to decompress when stimuli gets too intensive. The occupational therapist who has been working with a child can assist parents to organize a birthday party that is not too sensory intensive and that can be tolerated better.

Sensory Integrative Therapy for Early Childhood Mobility

The developing child learns to integrate balance (the vestibular system) with mobility to crawl and eventually walk. The vestibular system not only controls balance but also assists with integrating figure and ground, spatial relationships, and other sensory skills. In turn, these skills aid in the

Copyright © Mometrix Media. You have been licensed one copy of this document for personal use only. Any other reproduction or redistribution is strictly prohibited. All rights reserved.
This content is provided for test preparation purposes only and does not imply an endorsement by Mometrix of any particular political, scientific, or religious point of view.

ability to perform advanced movements such as running. Sensory integrative therapy aims to challenge balance and the vestibular system in a slow, methodical fashion. Activities such as swinging, rolling, and tumbling all challenge the vestibular system by increasing balance. Many times, sensory integrative therapy is referred to as play therapy as this is the primary occupation of children. Many times, children with sensory integrative problems are on the autistic spectrum. Mobility and autism work hand in hand. As the sensory integrative issues resolve, so do some of the autistic features.

Assisting Clients with Low Vision Maintain Engagement in Leisure Activities

People who develop low vision are often isolated and feel lonely. The occupational therapist (OT), through problem-solving techniques, is able to locate services, recommend home adaptations, and teach skills and strategies designed to improve the life of a client who has low vision. When engaging in a team approach, the OT can tap into resources such as an orientation mobility specialist, who can assist with the treatment of a person with low vision. Home adaptations, such as magnifiers for reading and marking home items with braille stickers, allow for the client to partake in tasks that otherwise would be inaccessible. Books on tape as well as text-to-speech software can assist the client in leisure tasks that were once enjoyable. Finally, special lighting can also assist with seeing objects that are not as visible to clients with low vision.

Compensatory Strategies for Managing Decreased Memory

Cognitive disabilities can be caused by developmental delay, stroke, traumatic brain injury, or some other pathology. Cognitive strategies have to be tailored to an individual's needs. One of the most common impairments is loss of memory. Computer drills that focus on memory as well as card games, visual imagery, and paragraph listening are approaches that have shown positive improvement in memory. Compensatory strategies include making lists, recording voice memos, and reducing outside stimuli. Frequent reminders by caregivers also serve to improve the recall of things such as lists, things to do, and times for events. Compensatory strategies are available to use on an as-needed basis. On better days, fewer strategies are necessary. However, on days the client is not feeling as well, compensatory strategies may be relied on heavily.

Remediation of Cognitive Deficits

Remediation means to restore lost function. Therefore, remediation of cognitive deficits aims to restore lost cognitive deficits when possible. There has to be a balance between remediation and compensation (finding alternative adaptive methods for doing a task). The length of time for remediation is not defined by days but determined by the accomplishment of goals. This can normally take several months (at least) to accomplish. Remedial cognitive tasks may involve memory or visual perceptual challenges that attempt to get the brain to redevelop the neural pathways to recover the lost function. These tasks can be exercises to develop better memory recall, visual perceptual games, and reading and auditory exercises for memory. Finally, remediation involves great patience and dedication on the part of the client and therapist.

Retraining Patients with Left Neglect

A precursor to visual scanning is the ability to attend to the left and right side of vision. Each hemisphere of the brain attends to visual attention. The left visual field is predominantly controlled by the right side of the brain and vice versa. However, most noticeable neglect occurs when the right side of the brain experiences damage and causes left neglect. Clients with neglect very seldom recover completely from this deficit. Instead, they are trained to compensate by turning their head to the side of neglect to begin to retrain the brain that both sides of the field of view exists. Patients are also retrained to attend to the left side of the body during activities of daily living (ADL) and

Copyright © Mometrix Media. You have been licensed one copy of this document for personal use only. Any other reproduction or redistribution is strictly prohibited. All rights reserved.
This content is provided for test preparation purposes only and does not imply an endorsement by Mometrix of any particular political, scientific, or religious point of view.

instrumental activities of daily living (IADL) tasks. Many times, patients with this type of neglect will need to have visual, auditory, or tactile cues to attend to the neglected side.

Receptive Aphasia

Receptive aphasia is a condition in which clients have difficulty understanding written or verbal language. This is exemplified by the patient not being able to respond appropriately or respond at all to verbal interaction. This is also referred to as Wernicke's aphasia. This type of aphasia refers to the area in the parietal lobe of the brain that contains one of the two centers for speech. Many of these patients do not have many, if any, motor deficits. Receptive aphasia is caused by damage in the brain such as a stroke. Treatment usually consists of speech therapy to work on cognitive skills, language skills, and linguistic skills. Finally, family members are trained to follow through with home programs as well as strategies for communicating with the patient.

Expressive Aphasia

This type of aphasia is also known as Broca's aphasia because of the area of the parietal lobe where expressive aphasia is originating. This type of aphasia results in the loss of the ability to vocalize thoughts. Sometimes speech is understood, but the sentence structure is incomplete. Other times, a client may speak in unintelligible words that are repetitive or have no meaning. Many times, these clients know what they want to express but just are not able to do so. Because these patients know what they want to communicate but are not able to do so, a high level of frustration is sometimes exhibited. Stroke is the most common cause of this type of aphasia. Treatment consists of word repetition and phrases as well as compensatory techniques lost language skills.

Global Aphasia

Global aphasia affects both Broca's area and Wernicke's areas of the brain. In other words, both receptive and expressive language is affected. Patients who are globally aphasic generally have a worse prognosis for recovery than those patients who are either receptive or expressive aphasic. Global aphasia generally results from occlusion of the middle cerebral artery. Improvements are best made when speech therapy is utilized. Therapy consists of learning how to gesture, pictures, and pointing to communicate. Therapy may be in a group setting or individual treatment sessions. People who try to communicate with these patients need to remember that it may take a longer period of time to form words or process incoming communication. Patience is very important.

Compensatory Techniques for Short-Term Memory Deficits

There are several effective techniques to improve short-term memory. It is easier to recall something if it is associated with something familiar. For instance, you can associate a date with an event or holiday that falls around the date you are trying to remember. Next, you can visualize what you are trying to remember. Another technique is to repeat new information several times. If necessary, break up the material into smaller parts. For instance, if you are trying to remember directions to someone's home, you can break up the directions into segments and concentrate on knowing one segment at a time. Finally, write things down. This is a sure way to remember information. Although the recovery of memory can improve with therapy, progress can be slow. Be sure to be patient with the client and offer encouragement.

Training People with Developmental Disabilities About Money Management Skills

Money management is an important life skill that occupational therapists assist clients in learning. Good budgeting and spending skills as well as discerning the difference between needs and wants are important to lay a good foundation for money management. Therapists assist in teaching instrumental activities of daily living (IADL) skills such as bill paying, grocery shopping, and

Copyright © Mometrix Media. You have been licensed one copy of this document for personal use only. Any other reproduction or redistribution is strictly prohibited. All rights reserved.
This content is provided for test preparation purposes only and does not imply an endorsement by Mometrix of any particular political, scientific, or religious point of view.

budgeting for leisure activities. The value of saving is taught as a skill for long-term planning. As clients earn and save money, they are taught how to interact with modern-day banking institutions as well as electronic interfaces such as ATM machines. It is necessary to train in methods to avoid identity theft. In the event of identification theft, clients need to know the sequence of steps necessary to report the loss as well as how to financially recover after this type of situation.

Educating the Client Undergoing Hip Replacement

It is normal for clients to feel apprehensive about hip surgery. Many people have lived with hip pain for a long time and are unsure if the outcomes of surgery will be successful. To train the new hip patient in precautions, safety, mobility, and activities of daily living (ADLs), many facilities will institute a pre-surgical hip group. This group meets prior to surgery and discusses what to expect post-surgery as well as introduces clients to precautions, equipment, and staff. Post-surgery, a course of rehab as well as thorough home assessment are important to give the patient a background that will lead to a successful transition from the hospital to home. The goal of any hip education program is to reduce the chance for falls. Fall hazards in the home must be assessed during the home evaluation and eliminated.

Adaptive Equipment for Patient on Lumbar Back Precautions After an L4-L5 Fusion

The important thing to remember is that lumbar back precautions means to not bend forward (from a sitting or standing position). Do not lift more than 10 lbs. Do not twist the trunk while performing an activity. Instead, turn the whole body toward the activity being performed. Do not cross knees or ankles as this places excessive strain on the low back. Finally, log roll out of bed instead of getting out of bed segmentally. The durable medical equipment most appropriate for this type of patient is a reacher for assisting to don or doff pants. A sock aid is useful to assist in donning socks. A long-handled shoehorn can aid in donning shoes, whereas a long-handled sponge can assist with bathing.

Oral Motor Skills

Oral motor development consists of the use and function of the lips, tongue, jaw, teeth, and hard and soft palates. The movement and coordination of these structures are important for swallowing liquids as well as consuming foods. Development of these structures occurs from prenatal stages to age three. The sequence of development is usually started pre-birth as the baby learns to suckle while in vitro. By 3 months, reflexes are established that protect the airway from choking. At 6 months, the baby is able to consume rice cereal and pureed fruit and vegetables. By 9 months, the baby is able to consume pureed meats. At 1 year, the baby is able to eat dissolvable solids such as crackers and small cereals. Finally, by 18 months, the baby is able to eat finely chopped table foods. It is not until 3 years that the baby is fully able to consume meats, fried foods, and whole fruits.

Oral Motor Compensatory Techniques for Eating

Just as the consistency of liquids can be altered to assist with swallowing, the consistency of foods can also be altered to assist with safe feeding. Foods can be chopped, minced, pureed, or liquified to assist with safe feeding. Additionally, the patient should be encouraged to sit upright during the meal as well as 30 minutes after the meal. This allows time for food to be digested enough to prevent reflux and aspiration of food into the lungs. It is important to allow extra time for feeding and to encourage the patient to pause between mouthfuls to allow the complete swallowing of foods prior to the next bite. Sometimes eating three times daily is too fatiguing. In this case large meals may be broken up into several smaller meals throughout the day.

Copyright © Mometrix Media. You have been licensed one copy of this document for personal use only. Any other reproduction or redistribution is strictly prohibited. All rights reserved.
This content is provided for test preparation purposes only and does not imply an endorsement by Mometrix of any particular political, scientific, or religious point of view.

Oral Motor Techniques to Facilitate Swallowing

It is important to realize that proper body alignment is necessary for safe swallowing. A neutral alignment of the pelvis allows the spine and head to align properly for swallowing. The shoulders should be held back and head aligned over the cervical spine. There are two types of exercises for dysphasia—indirect and direct exercise. Exercise is generally aimed at increasing range of motion, coordination, and strength of the jaw, lips, cheek, tongue, soft palate, and vocal cords. Head lift exercises increase the opening of the esophageal sphincter. Exercises to strengthen lip muscles, such as blowing through a straw, as well as tongue-strengthening exercises work to enforce the oral motor phase of swallowing. Electrical stimulation is applied to the neck area to also facilitate later phases of swallowing.

Compensatory Techniques to Safely Swallow Liquids After a Stroke

Liquid textures may need to be altered after a stroke to allow for safe swallowing. There are four types of textures for liquids. Level one is slightly thick. Level two is mildly thick. Level three is moderately thick. Finally, level four is extremely thick. Liquids are thickened with a starch-based thickener based upon radiographic studies and a speech pathologist's recommendations. Clients should also use strategies such as sitting upright, taking small sips, keeping the chin slightly tucked, avoiding talking during drinking, and reducing distractions. Even though liquids may be thickened, it is important to drink six to eight cups of liquid daily. If the patient exhibits signs and symptoms of dysphagia, allow him or her to rest prior to drinking more fluid. Always allow an extended period of time to consume liquids.

Dysphagia

Dysphagia can lead to aspiration pneumonia as foods and liquids are often routed to the lungs instead of the esophagus. People who have aspirated will often show symptoms such as coughing, wheezing, and mucous/saliva mixed secretions in the mouth. There are, however, a group of people who show no signs and symptoms of aspiration. This is a condition referred to as silent aspiration. Silent aspiration has no symptoms until the day pneumonia sets into the lungs. Patients who have risks for silent aspiration are identified with a radiographic study called a modified barium swallow test. To avoid silent aspiration, bedbound patients need to have the head of the bed elevated as close to 30 degrees as possible. It is best not to lie down for 30 to 45 minutes after mealtime.

Ideal Mealtime Environment When Facilitating Oral Motor Skills

There are several key concepts that need to be taught to the client as well as caregivers to encourage a safe dining environment during meals. It is important to create a relaxed dining environment as tension of any muscle group can cause swallowing difficulties. It is also important to minimize distractions. Good oral hygiene also helps with the chewing process, which in turn, helps alleviate un-chewed food due to painful gums and teeth. The presentation of food to the patient should take into consideration factors such as neglect, visual deficits, and motor ability to use utensils. Some clients may also require the plate or bowl to be placed to one side or the other depending upon neglect as well as the affected side. Finally, ensure the food remains warm throughout the meal as, many times, consistency is affected by temperature.

Caregiver's Responsibility in Facilitating Oral Motor Skills

The main job of the caregiver is to ensure the safe eating and drinking of the patient. It is important for the patient with dysphagia to have a quiet place to dine. This helps eliminate distractions. The caregiver should also be encouraged to partake in family training to learn which techniques and cues are required to assist the patient in eating and drinking. Once strategies are learned, they should consistently be followed. Tips for cooking include cooking meat until tender, cooking

Copyright © Mometrix Media. You have been licensed one copy of this document for personal use only. Any other reproduction or redistribution is strictly prohibited. All rights reserved.
This content is provided for test preparation purposes only and does not imply an endorsement by Mometrix of any particular political, scientific, or religious point of view.

vegetables in water to ensure softness, making mashed potatoes lump free, and removing seeds, husks, skins, and gristle. Finally, it is important for the caregiver to learn cardiopulmonary resuscitation. If a client chokes during a meal, the caregiver has a period of minutes to perform a rescue and prevent injury.

PREVOCATIONAL, VOCATIONAL, AND TRANSITIONAL SERVICES

Prevocational services are those that prepare people with disabilities for jobs that pay and help them achieve greater independence in their communities. Prevocational services teach job skills and concepts rather than specific work skills for a particular job. Vocational services, however, teach specific skills for specific job settings. Often, standardized tests are used to identify strengths and possible vocations. Transitional services go beyond vocational services in that they prepare an individual to be part of a community. These services aim not only to develop work-related skills but to foster living skills such as activities of daily living (ADLs), instrumental activities of daily living (IADLs), and social integration into the community. Transitional services may incorporate other disciplines to reach an end goal set by the patient, patient's family, and care team.

PREVOCATIONAL SERVICES

Prevocational services are often used with people with developmental disabilities. These services include training in basic skills such as following directions, attending to task, task completion, problem-solving, and safety. These services are provided to clients who are not expected to join the work force in one year. Prevocational services also train in the use of technology, service delivery, assess for work interests; provide training in the use of public transportation and in the concepts of job performance and performance requirements; and assist the individual develop appropriate attitudes, behaviors, and workplace habits. These services are customarily provided in the most integrated setting. Simulated workplaces are good environments to begin prevocational training. It is for this reason that many day programs incorporate prevocational services into their daily routines.

VOCATIONAL SERVICES

The goal of vocational services is to assist the individual (usually with developmental disabilities) hold a job of choice within the community. The interest and capabilities of each person is assessed, and jobs with suitable technical and social skills are matched to the individual's strengths. Many individuals in this type of program are paired with job coaches who provide customized on-site support, including transportation, job training, and oversight. Often small group training is used to train individuals in the employment skills of punctuality, personal hygiene, workplace etiquette, time management, self-control, stress management, and using public transportation. States often fund vocational services for individuals with developmental disabilities. Many vocational programs offer a small stipend so that clients begin to learn the value of money. Graduates of this program often go on to meaningful vocations as well as work their way up the vocational ladder to become managers.

TRANSITIONAL SERVICES

Often, individuals with intellectual and developmental disabilities are ready to move into a more independent living situation. Transitional services are designed to bridge the gap between one living and vocational setting into another. For many, this transition may mean moving from a group home situation into an apartment in which the individual is living on his or her own. Transitional services not only train the client in self-care skills and work skills but also in household tasks, looking for employment, shopping, money management, accessing transportation, health and wellness, and skill development. A major goal of transitional services is to make sure each

Copyright © Mometrix Media. You have been licensed one copy of this document for personal use only. Any other reproduction or redistribution is strictly prohibited. All rights reserved.
This content is provided for test preparation purposes only and does not imply an endorsement by Mometrix of any particular political, scientific, or religious point of view.

individual is confident in his or her abilities. Such confidence is often developed prior to individuals moving to live on their own by developing routines and skills for independent living.

Vocational Assessment Process for Individuals with Disabilities

The assessment process for individuals with disabilities makes use of the same materials as in the school, employment service, and psychological settings. Sometimes, the procedures for testing are adapted to persons with disabilities. The assessment process focuses on identifying abilities and strengths that can be used in training and work situations. The assessment process may contain an interview with a vocational officer, examination of work and school records, medical exam, appropriate aptitude tests, technical or trade tests, and analysis of physical capabilities. These tests may be carried out by a multidisciplinary team including therapists, doctors, social workers, and vocational specialists. Overall the assessment is conducted through interviews, standardized tests, observation, and review of background information. Once the assessment process is complete and recommendations are made, an interdisciplinary conference is held with the client and family to discuss findings and decide a path forward.

Occupational Therapist's Role in Transitional Home Setting

Adults in transitional settings face many challenges. Many of these people have mental and physical disabilities. Some people may have even come from homeless situations. It is important to assess activities of daily living (ADL) skills to determine a client's ability to perform expected daily care. Instrumental activities of daily living (IADL) skills are also assessed to determine potential for vocational placement. The occupational therapist (OT) also makes recommendations for involvement in community volunteer activities. Necessary skills are determined and worked on during therapy sessions. Carryover into the home setting is important as skill attainment can take months to accomplish. Tasks within the home are assigned to clients based upon ability, preference, and necessary skill attainment for future employment. Payment for tasks may come as monetary compensation or as privileges within the home. Finally, the OT may assess for needed adaptive equipment for the home setting as well as vocational settings.

Medical Alert

The medical alert is a good way for medically fragile people and older adults to have access to emergency services if they should fall, do not feel well, or are in any type of emergency. The medical alert is used by pushing a button that directly calls 911 (some medical alerts have the option of calling phone numbers prior to calling 911). Most medical alerts can reach at least a few hundred yards. However, the wireless medical alert runs on a cellular service and can be used anywhere a cell phone is able to operate. The medical alert is not for everyone; those people with cognitive deficits may have difficulty remembering to wear or use a medical alert.

Transferring from Bed to Wheelchair for Lower Extremity Amputees

Lower extremity amputee patients run the risk of falls. When transferring from the bed to a wheelchair, it is important to enact several safety steps. First, try to get the chair and bed on the same level so that transfers are straight across instead of at a different height. If a stand pivot transfer is too difficult, a sliding board transfer may be more appropriate. Make sure there is a stable object (such as a portable bed rail) to hold onto when performing the transfer. Finally, make sure the armrest of the wheelchair (on the side of the transfer) is raised to allow an unencumbered transfer. Occasionally a patient may become dizzy when coming from supine to sitting. In this case, have the patient sit on the edge of the bed until the dizziness has receded.

Copyright © Mometrix Media. You have been licensed one copy of this document for personal use only. Any other reproduction or redistribution is strictly prohibited. All rights reserved.
This content is provided for test preparation purposes only and does not imply an endorsement by Mometrix of any particular political, scientific, or religious point of view.

TLSO

The occupational therapist's (OT's) role with the patient with a thoracic-lumbar-sacral orthosis (TLSO) is one of education. The patient should be taught how to don and doff the TLSO as well as how to maintain hygiene. The TLSO should be worn at all times when out of bed. That means that prior to transferring out of bed, the client is taught how to don and doff the device while in the supine position. Precautions for this device also involve no twisting or bending while wearing the device. This is a good time for the OT to review proper body mechanics with the patient to prevent future injury. The TLSO is maintained by taking off the pads, which are attached by Velcro, and wiping down the inside of the shell with a moist, soapy towel. The pads may be hand washed in warm water and air dried.

Assistance of OT in Wellness Program for Diabetes

Occupational therapists (OTs) can educate and teach clients to modify eating habits and include exercise to lead healthier lifestyles. OTs can also teach how to monitor calorie and sugar intake. Meal planning and preparation as well as exercise are good activities for OTs to incorporate into treatment plans. Cooking activities can focus on healthy food preparation as well as portion control. Exercise should incorporate strengthening as well as aerobic qualities. For those individuals with disabilities such as low vision, sensory loss in hands and fine motor loss, occupational therapy can train in compensatory techniques for vision using adaptive equipment as well as fine motor skills and related adaptive equipment. Medication pill boxes and auditory/visual reminders may have to be used to accommodate the scheduled taking of medications.

Implementing a Heart Healthy Diet into Cooking Activity

A cooking activity for a patient that requires a heart-healthy diet needs to begin with meal preparation. Actively involve the client in preparing foods he or she enjoys eating and may be able to prepare using heart-healthy ingredients. Teach the importance of eating vegetables and fruits. Also teach the value of portion control. Suggest the substitution of whole grains instead of enriched flour. As the client prepares a meal, emphasize using low-fat and non-saturated fat foods and oils. Finally, substitute herbs for salt when possible. A cooking activity will demonstrate that healthy cooking can be tasty as well as quick. There are many healthy recipe books (e.g., Weight Watchers) that allow for the cooking of quick but tasty meals. It is also important to plan a sample menu of all meals with the client to provide an example of how each meal might be prepared using heart-healthy principles.

Slowing Age-Related Cardiopulmonary Changes

A combination of a heart-healthy diet, low stress, exercise, and sleep are all important to maintaining cardiopulmonary health. Diet includes staying away from saturated and trans fats, such as red meat, high-fat dairy products, and fried foods. Fats containing omega-3 fatty acids lower triglyceride levels and can be found in products such as fish. Exercise should never be started without a doctor's approval. Good forms of exercise involve an aerobic workout such as walking, jogging, swimming, or biking. The American Heart Association recommends 150 minutes of moderate exercise or 75 minutes of strenuous exercise per week. This can be divided into two segments per day and/or three to five times per week. Finally, lack of sleep contributes to coronary artery calcification, hypertension, and diabetes, heart attack, and stroke.

Copyright © Mometrix Media. You have been licensed one copy of this document for personal use only. Any other reproduction or redistribution is strictly prohibited. All rights reserved.
This content is provided for test preparation purposes only and does not imply an endorsement by Mometrix of any particular political, scientific, or religious point of view.

Improving Sensory, Motor, Neurological, and Physiological Status

Grading for Therapeutic Exercise and Conditioning Programs

After an evaluation, the occupational therapist determines long- and short-term goals. The method from getting from the short- to long-term goals is often defined as the way to grade an activity. Therapeutic exercise consists of things such as TheraBands, free weights, weight machines, exercise cycles, and walking, jogging, and running activities. Grading can come in the form of making a physical activity more difficult by adding things like weights and/or repetitions. Grading for therapeutic exercise considers the factors of age, diagnosis, and premorbid status. Grading occurs in a slow manner when muscle recovery as well as recovery from illness is concerned. Always confer with the ordering physician as well as any other relevant care providers to ensure the exercise and conditioning program is properly designed for the patient.

TheraBand

TheraBand exercises use an elastic resistance band. The resistance of the band is dependent upon the amount of stretch given to the band. TheraBands are color coded with resistance increasing from least to most as follows: tan, yellow, red, green, blue, black, silver, and gold. TheraBands can be used to exercise the upper and lower body. There are precautions and contraindications for using TheraBands. TheraBand exercises should not be used with patients who have had recent thoracic surgery. Patients who have significant upper body pain should also avoid TheraBand exercises as pressure on joints can exacerbate pain and arthritis. TheraBands should be started slowly, at first, with few repetitions. As repetitions are increased consider moving to the next color of TheraBand. Muscle pain that is persistent is an indication that progression of exercise is too quick.

Grading a Cardiac Rehabilitation Program

Cardiac rehab orders for a client usually come with specific parameters that physicians want therapists to follow during exercise. Target heart rates are closely monitored as well as oxygen saturation and blood pressure. Once the target heart rate for exercise is reached with decreasing effort, consider upgrading the program. This can be done with more repetitions or increasing the intensity of exercise. Additionally, another sign that it is time to upgrade the cardiac program is when clients state they are not pushing themselves to complete the exercise. Any exercise that involves weight should allow for 6 to 12 repetitions prior to fatigue. Over time, blood pressure as well as heart rate will decrease with exercise. Decreased resting heart is also a good sign of physical fitness.

Grading Active Assistive Range of Motion Activities

Active assistive range of motion movements are partially done by the patient and partially assisted by a device or therapist. For instance, overhead pulleys are a good active assisted exercise to increase shoulder motion. However, as with all active assistive exercise, do not increase range of motion beyond the point of comfort. Assistive range of motion should be performed in a moderately slow fashion to maintain pain-free motion. A slow, prolonged stretch is also recommended to allow muscle fibers time to relax. Orthopedic patients should have specific parameters for increasing range of motion as per the physician's protocol. When increasing range of motion, it is often helpful to apply heat prior to exercise to warm up tissues and cold post exercise is to decrease inflammation caused by exercise.

Grading Passive Range of Motion Activities

Passive range of motion is motion completed for the patient by someone else. Passive range of motion may be performed on stroke patients as a way to maintain joint and muscle integrity as well

Copyright © Mometrix Media. You have been licensed one copy of this document for personal use only. Any other reproduction or redistribution is strictly prohibited. All rights reserved.
This content is provided for test preparation purposes only and does not imply an endorsement by Mometrix of any particular political, scientific, or religious point of view.

as orthopedic patients who have had recent trauma or surgery. Slow, rhythmical motion is the standard for performing passive range of motion. Do not go beyond the point of comfort for the patient. Because the patient is not able to assist in the motion of the joint, it is important to pay attention to the end feel of the joint, the patient's verbal and nonverbal communication, and physician's orders. Family members who are taught passive range of motion exercises should be able to demonstrate proper handling techniques for the occupational therapist. Apply heat prior to exercise to warm up tissues and cold post exercise to decrease inflammation caused by exercise.

Grading an Exercise Performed on Exercise Cycles

It is important to be aware that exercise cycles should not be a substitute for skilled therapy. Exercise cycles are good for restorative care but should be limited in the clinic setting. That being said, exercise cycles are used to build endurance. All patients, especially cardiac-involved patients, should have vital signs checked and monitored prior, during, and after exercise. Most exercise cycles allow for the grading of resistance as well as speed. When grading this activity, it is better to increase speed and endurance separately from each other to identify which factor is most useful or is causing any ill effects. Patients with lower endurance may benefit from occasional rest breaks. Like speed and resistance, the frequency of rest breaks can also be graded.

Safety Procedures for Using TheraBands

TheraBands are a common exercise tool used in most therapy settings. However, there have been numerous reports of eye injuries associated with TheraBands due to the band breaking and striking the eye. Due to the therapeutic use of TheraBands, the benefits of its use outweigh the risk of injury. That being said, there are a few important precautions to observe. First, use the band in a plane that does not risk hitting yourself or anyone else if it should break. Second, inspect the band prior to use to look for worn or torn areas on the band. Discard the band if any defective areas are found, and start with a fresh piece of TheraBand for exercise. Finally, store the band in a cool, dry place that avoids direct sunlight or heat.

Implementing an HEP with a Client Who is Ambivalent to Exercise

The home exercise program (HEP) is not designed to make Olympic athletes. Instead, the HEP is intended to carry over (and progress) the gains made in therapy into the home setting. Occupational therapy is not intended to last indefinitely. The client and family should be adequately trained to perform the HEP on their own once discharged from therapy. The rewards for continuing the HEP are the abilities that the client gains and carries over into functional tasks. For instance, the increase in hand strength and dexterity after stroke therapy can be used to encourage self-feeding and the resumption of hobbies. Praise the client for any gains made. Encourage functional activity along with the HEP. Incorporate functional activities in the HEP as a way of breaking up the monotony. Finally, plan on incorporate a rest of one or two days each week from the HEP.

Home Exercise Program to Increase Finger Flexion Post Carpal Tunnel Surgery

A home program post carpal tunnel surgery consists of extensor tendon gliding and median nerve gliding exercises. All exercises should be done slowly and held for 15 to 30 seconds. These can be repeated three to five times each as tolerated. First, with wrist in neutral position, bend all of the fingers to make a fist and hold. Second, open fingers and extend thumb upward and hold. Third, extend fingers and wrist upward from the neutral position. Keep thumb at the side of the fingers. Third, bend fingers at knuckles only while keeping distal finger joints straight. The fourth exercise involves bending knuckles and the first distal joint while keeping the second distal joint straight. Finally, with all fingers and thumb together, laterally bend wrist to left and right side.

Copyright © Mometrix Media. You have been licensed one copy of this document for personal use only. Any other reproduction or redistribution is strictly prohibited. All rights reserved.
This content is provided for test preparation purposes only and does not imply an endorsement by Mometrix of any particular political, scientific, or religious point of view.

Precautions for Orders for Range of Motion After Reduction of the Right Shoulder

A patient who has just had a reduction of the right shoulder after a dislocation comes to your clinic and has orders for range of motion. Unfortunately, you will see vague orders like this frequently. It is difficult to plan treatment around these orders as there are no notes indicating whether the dislocation was anterior or posterior, stability of the joint, previous medical history, and physician's protocol. Orders such as this can do more harm than good if the therapist is not familiar with the diagnosis. It is also essential to know the history of the present illness. Information such as the activity performed when the injury occurred, work responsibilities, leisure interests, and home responsibilities are all part of the picture that defines the patient. Premorbid status is also a good way to determine what the patient may want to achieve post-therapy. It is always good to have as much of this information prior to the patient arriving for the first day of therapy. Office staff can be of good assistance in retrieving this information for therapy staff.

Precautions After Right Total Hip Replacement Due to Pathological Fracture in Cancer Patient

Pathological fractures happen as a result of a disease process, in this case, cancer. The bone and joint are likely to have weakened due to a cancerous process within the hip or femur. It will be important to look at X-rays as well as have the physician determine if there is a malignancy in the bone or joint and where the malignancy is located. This patient will have the same hip precautions as a regular hip replacement. However, there will likely be the addition of weight-bearing precautions for a few weeks to give the bone a chance to heal without the stress of weight. Strict adherence to not bending over 90 degrees as well as no external rotation of the hip will be important as this new hip will likely dislocate easier than a non-pathological hip.

Expected Functional Performance of a C5 Quadriplegic

The level of C5 corresponds with motor loss to hands, triceps, partial biceps, as well as partial shoulder. Patients with C5 quadriplegia may be able to lift their shoulders to about 90 degrees against gravity. Partial bicep flexion assists the wrist with extension to close the hand in a Tenodesis movement. This movement is useful for holding objects in the hand such as a sandwich and built-up handles for brushing teeth and hair. Most feeding is done through finger foods. A universal cuff is also useful to assist in the eating of foods requiring a spoon. Most self-care is performed with the assistance of others. A universal cuff may also be used to perform instrumental activities of daily living (IADLs) such as typing (with a stylus). Adaptive equipment is often added to phones, power wheelchairs, and vehicles.

Role of NDT in Recovery of Stroke Patients

The goal of Neurodevelopmental Treatment (NDT) is to promote motor learning through patient participation in functional tasks and simulated tasks. Evaluation posture and movements are looked at for abnormalities that present during functional movement. Through handling, facilitation of movement, and activating key points of control, the client gradually relearns the motor sequence required for normal movement. Normal movements are then incorporated into functional tasks. Frequently, the inhibition of abnormal movement is also a consideration during treatment. The underlying premise for this treatment is that the brain has the capabilities, through plasticity, to develop new neural pathways that can override damaged ones. NDT theorists maintain that stroke recovery is a process that occurs through active follow-through of therapy when the patient is at home. Family members are a crucial part in assisting the patient to participate in a home program.

Copyright © Mometrix Media. You have been licensed one copy of this document for personal use only. Any other reproduction or redistribution is strictly prohibited. All rights reserved.
This content is provided for test preparation purposes only and does not imply an endorsement by Mometrix of any particular political, scientific, or religious point of view.

Faciliatory Techniques for Low Muscle Tone in Stroke Patients

Low muscle tone can be caused by stroke or traumatic brain injury (TBI) in adults. The faciliatory techniques remain the same for low muscle tone in stroke as well as TBI. To facilitate tone, you want to increase neural activity. The common facilitatory techniques are used to increase stimulation to the proprioceptive, vestibular, special senses (vision, hearing, taste, and smell) and autonomic systems. The techniques of vibration, tapping the muscle, brushing, icing, and manual contact are used to increase tone. Bearing weight through a joint is also a good method to increase the feedback loop from the joint and muscle to the brain. Passive as well as active assisted movements in all planes assist the proprioceptive system to relearn where the joint is in relation to space. It is important for the patient to also practice self-range of motion exercises throughout the day.

Sensory Reeducation

Sensory reeducation can refer to either a nerve or neurologic injury (such as stroke). With a nerve injury, there are generally two phases of recovery. In the early phase, the repaired nerve is trained to tolerate moving and constant touch. The late phase of reeducation focuses on finer touch for discerning objects and recognizing textures. In a stroke, sensory pathways are retrained to regulate over- or under-sensitive responses to touch. Many times, touch is absent or unrecognizable to the patient due to neural pathway injury. The goal is to facilitate feeling and recognition of objects. This directly impacts the functional use of the hand for fine motor activities. Safety is also affected in the absence of hot and cold discrimination. A method to compensate for loss of sensation is an equally important goal.

Motor Reeducation

Motor reeducation refers to training the neurologic system to perform normal movement after a brain injury from a stroke or traumatic brain injury. An evaluation must incorporate some form of movement analysis as well as assessment of activities of daily living (ADLs). The components of cognition, range of motion, sensation, strength, tone, synergistic movements, and adaptability are assessed. With the assistance of the client, goals are set. Motor relearning involves practice, feedback from the neurologic system, as well as the therapist. The more the patient experiences assisted movement in a normal fashion, the more the neurologic system will be retrained to perform normal movement unassisted. As with most therapy, it is important for a home program to be assigned and explained to available caregivers. Some form of range of motion (self-range of motion preferred) is important to incorporate as part of the home program.

Pain Management

Pain affects the performance of activities. The goal of therapy is to have patients participate in activities that have value and meaning to them. Strategies such as activity management, activity adaptation, developing coping strategies, and vocational rehab are all incorporated into the program for the client. Therapy may take place in a workplace, clinic, hospital, or patient's home. As clients with chronic pain often exhibit signs of depression, the occupational therapy is vital to determine which activities can be performed (adapted) by the patient while eliciting as little pain as possible. Biofeedback is often used in conjunction with an activity and/or exercise to give the client information to reduce muscle tension during performed activities/exercises. Progression is often one tool used to combat muscle tension as it attunes the patient to the stress in concentrated parts of the body.

Copyright © Mometrix Media. You have been licensed one copy of this document for personal use only. Any other reproduction or redistribution is strictly prohibited. All rights reserved.
This content is provided for test preparation purposes only and does not imply an endorsement by Mometrix of any particular political, scientific, or religious point of view.

Desensitizing the Hand to Touch

The desensitization program for the hand is aimed at improving feeling in the hand and therefore increase hand function. Exercises are performed two to three times daily for 10 minutes. Beginning with a smooth texture (such as a cotton ball), lightly rub the sensitive area for up to 10 minutes. When the texture is tolerated, move to a rougher texture. The order of progression should be cotton to flannel to denim to corduroy. Finally, tapping and vibration can be added. The occupational therapist is free to interject other textures into any part of the program. Progress is made when a texture is no longer noxious. It is very important to remain consistent in the implementation of this program as the outcome will come sooner with diligence.

Reducing Upper Extremity Edema

The occupational therapy includes edema as part of a standard evaluation. Measurements are taken prior to treatment. Motion and muscle strength help determine the effect of edema on function. The patient is taught to elevate the extremity to allow gravity to eliminate the edema. Massage is also used to encourage lymphatic return of fluids from the extremity to the circulatory system. Massage is always started at the distal extremity and worked downward toward the body. Exercise is also encouraged as it assists in recovering the function of the pumps and valves within vessels, which encourages the steady flow of bodily fluids. Many times, the physician will prescribe compression garments to be worn in conjunction with therapy.

Scar Management

Scarring can cause reduced range of motion and strength as well as increased pain. Additionally, scars pose the risk of keloid formation, adhesions, and infection. As a result, the performance of activities of daily living (ADLs) is negatively affected. Occupational therapists work to reduce scars and their impact through scar massage, compression therapy such as pressure garments, topical gels, splinting or casting, and desensitization. Any equipment needs are addressed to encourage maximal functional status during the healing process. Active exercises are important to increase range of motion, strength, and activity tolerance with a natural method. Ultrasound is also is used as a method to soften and reduce the size of a scar. Finally, the client is trained on a home program that contains the components of stretch, range of motion, massage, and strengthening.

Postural Stability

Postural stability involves the ability to control core muscles to sit or stand upright without leaning to one side or falling. Diseases that affect the neurologic system as well as orthopedic problems (such as scoliosis) affect postural control. The goal of therapy is to regain postural control to participate in purposeful activities. Postural control allows the upper body to position itself in space and provide purposeful movement to perform tasks such as reaching and lifting objects without losing balance. The stability of the torso also allows for movements in any plane to allow for pushing, pulling, and lifting. Postural stability is also important when eating food as alignment of the digestive system is important to swallow food without chocking as well as digest food properly.

Dynamic Balance

Dynamic balance is the body's ability to anticipate and react to changes in balance as the body moves in space. Dynamic balance is used during sitting tasks (e.g., tying shoes or donning pants) as well as standing tasks (e.g., laundry or washing a car). Dynamic balance activities can be graded based upon the client's level of function. Basic activities can include things such as sitting to stack cones or catching a ball (sitting or standing). Activities can progress to advanced tasks such as side stepping over the side of a tub or shower, sitting and standing from a toilet, and retrieving dishes from a shelf or dishwasher. The occupational therapist can also practice dynamic activities for

Copyright © Mometrix Media. You have been licensed one copy of this document for personal use only. Any other reproduction or redistribution is strictly prohibited. All rights reserved.
This content is provided for test preparation purposes only and does not imply an endorsement by Mometrix of any particular political, scientific, or religious point of view.

leisure skills such as horseshoes, table tennis, and golf. Nintendo Wii games also offer a good, fun platform for practicing dynamic balance skills.

Proper Body Mechanics for Lifting Objects from the Floor

Proper body mechanics serves three purposes. First, it ensures client safety. Second, proper body mechanics places less strain on the back (especially low back). Finally, proper body mechanics help conserve energy. When lifting an object from the floor, use knees to bend down and pick up the object. Keep the object close to the body to maintain a close center of gravity. It is also helpful to widen your base of support by opening your legs. When lifting the object, keep it close to the body as you straighten your knees. Avoid twisting when placing an object. Instead, turn and place the object. When possible, push, pull, roll, or slide an object instead of lifting it.

Proper Body Mechanics for Lifting Objects Overhead

The principles of lifting an object overhead are the same as lifting an object from floor level. It is important to keep the center of gravity toward your body. It is wise to not place objects above shoulder height. However, in cases in which it is necessary to place objects above shoulder height, it is important to use your arms to lift the object overhead. Make sure you walk directly in front of the object. Turn—do not twist to place the object in its resting place. Sometimes, a step stool can be safely used to lift an object overhead without overextending the spine. Slide the object on the shelf. A word of caution—repeated lifting of objects overhead is not good for the shoulders and can cause pain.

Efficient Breathing for Activities

Most people will hold their breath while lifting or doing strenuous activity. Holding your breath increases pressure inside the chest, which can, in turn, impede blood flow to the heart as well as raise blood pressure. A much healthier way of breathing during exercise is to learn to slowly blow out air during the exertion part of the exercise. For instance, when lifting a weight, teach patients to breathe in through the nose prior to the exercise. Let the air out slowly as the weight is lifted. Repeat during each repetition of the exercise. Breathing should be done in a slow, rhythmical fashion. This will also serve to regulate the pace of repetitions. Ensuring proper posture techniques will also enhance and ease breathing. Exercises such as yoga also feature proper breathing techniques and are good for flexibility as well.

Activities to Increase Balance Needed to Tie a Shoe

The type of balance described in this activity is dynamic sitting balance. First, perform a test of static sitting balance to assess basic stability. If basic stability is good, dynamic balance activities can be the focus of treatment. From a mat level, exercises such as stacking cones from different heights, batting a balloon, forward reaching, and overhead reaching can be performed first. As balance increases, incorporate tying shoes into the activity. Either crossing one knee over the other or bending to tie the shoes can be attempted. However, keep the mat level where the client's feet can touch the floor. Adaptive elastic shoe laces that require no tying can be used to compensate for lack of balance in cases in which the patient is expected to tie the shoe on his or her own.

Osteoarthritis and Gardening

People with osteoarthritis typically present with joint swelling, pain, and redness. Additionally, stiffness often limits range of motion as well as strength. Activities, such as gardening, can be performed but in a modified fashion. Although bending at the knees and activities at ground level are unsafe for these clients, planters can be placed on tables at wheelchair or standing level. Standing or sitting while performing this activity is a modification to increase safety, by reducing

Copyright © Mometrix Media. You have been licensed one copy of this document for personal use only. Any other reproduction or redistribution is strictly prohibited. All rights reserved.
This content is provided for test preparation purposes only and does not imply an endorsement by Mometrix of any particular political, scientific, or religious point of view.

the chance for falls, as well as a modification to reduce knee pain. Tools used in this activity need to have large or built-up handles. Finally, work height should be between the waist and shoulder.

Using Orthotic and Prosthetic Devices to Support Functional Outcomes

Joint Mobilization

Joint mobilization is the use of a skilled graded force to move a joint in a desired direction. Unlike stretching a muscle, joint mobilization is specific to the joint capsule. The technique to perform joint mobilization involves gliding of the joint with the therapist's hands in a specified direction. Occupational therapists (OTs) most commonly perform joint mobilization on the shoulder, wrist, and hand. Most joints that require hands on are stiff due to lack of motion from injury or surgery. The person is placed in a position of comfort that allows the joint that will be mobilized to move freely. The OT uses hands to gradually apply increased pressure over the joint (sometimes in conjunction with oscillation) in the desired direction. It may take several sessions for the patient to tolerate increased pressure and oscillations. However, with time, as motion is increased, a transition to active movements of the joint is incorporated into treatments.

Immobilization

Immobilization is the process of placing a bone and/or joint in a splint, brace, or cast to prevent injury during the healing process. Casts are generally used to immobilize broken bones. Splints are used to immobilize a dislocated joint as it heals. Splints are often used on the wrist, hand, and fingers. Splints can be used to immobilize for healing as well as for positioning. Splints that are used for positioning are either soft splints in the form of foam or hard splints made from a plastic material called Thermoplast. Thermoplastic materials are pliable when heated and conform to molded positions when cooled. Immobilization for fractures needs to follow strict a strict protocol as prescribed by an orthopedic surgeon. However, splinting for positioning, although needing a doctor's prescription, follows occupational therapy protocols.

Occupational Therapy Assistant's Role in Splint Fabrication

Splints can be fabricated by either occupational therapists (OTs) or OT assistants. Although both OTs and OT assistants are clinically trained, OT assistants get a slight bit more clinical experience as they have less involvement in the evaluation process. OTs are primarily involved in evaluations (in most clinics). As such, that leaves the OT assistant to perform the treatments and complete splint fabrication. It is a good idea for the OT to include splint fabrication in the assistant's performance competencies if the work environment involves splinting on a regular basis. This allows the OT to confirm and document the performance competency of the OT assistant during the splinting process. The assistant must give special consideration to any questions regarding the splint process as appropriate.

Considerations for Splinting

There are several objectives to splinting. First is to prevent contractures by reducing spasticity. This is best achieved during the course of a 12- to 16-week period. The second objective is to protect after injury or surgery. During the post-operative phase of treatment, a dynamic splint may be prescribed if the doctor indicates he or she wants to allow for movement. Otherwise, a static splint is prescribed. The third reason for splinting is to progressively stretch tissues. This is done in the case of burns, early stages of contractures, and post-surgery. Splinting is usually not done over open wounds, bruises, or hypersensitivity. The skin must always be inspected for red areas prior to

Copyright © Mometrix Media. You have been licensed one copy of this document for personal use only. Any other reproduction or redistribution is strictly prohibited. All rights reserved.
This content is provided for test preparation purposes only and does not imply an endorsement by Mometrix of any particular political, scientific, or religious point of view.

and post-splinting. Red areas lasting more than 20 minutes mean the splint needs to be adjusted so that it is not rubbing the area.

Dynamic Splinting

Dynamic splinting stretches joints that are lacking in motion. The goal of dynamic splinting is to stress scarred or shortened connective tissue to promote nontraumatic and more permanent tissue remodeling. When tissues are elongated, range of motion is increased. A dynamic splint consists of a thermoplastic splint with metal moveable parts that are connected to one or more joints. A constant load is placed on the desired joint(s) through the use of rubber bands. The amount of tension is regulated by the angle of pull as well as rubber band length. Normally, dynamic splints are worn, initially, for an hour. As the splint is tolerated, increased wear time is encouraged. Wear time can build up to two to three hours to several hours daily. These types of splints are most often used for trauma, joint replacements, ligament or tendon repairs, long-term immobilization, and joint stiffness.

Static Splints Versus Dynamic Splints

Static splints are good to use in some instances but not all cases. Static splints are best used to prevent deformities from tone, to immobilize a joint when it has been broken, to reduce tone, and to rest soft tissue surrounding the joints of the wrist and hand. The disadvantage of static splinting is that it can cause joint stiffness. Dynamic splints are best used when certain movements to a joint are allowed but other movements are restricted. The advantage of dynamic splinting is that it helps prevent joint stiffness. The disadvantage to this type of splint is that the more complicated splints with outriggers are very complex and must have precise placement of the outrigger to allow for the proper pull angle of pull on tendons.

Resting Hand Splint

The resting hand splint can be used to reduce pain and swelling, protect inflamed joints of the hand, and provide proper positioning during sleep. Patients with the diagnosis of stroke, tenosynovitis, carpal tunnel syndrome, osteoarthritis, or rheumatoid arthritis commonly are prescribed this type of splint. Proper positioning for a resting hand splint involves the wrist at 10 to 15 degrees of extension, the metacarpal phalanges at 15 to 20 degrees of flexion, the proximal inter-phalanges joints at 20 to 25 degrees of flexion, and the distal inter-phalanges at 10 degrees flexion. The splint is worn for 1 to 2 hours at first and gradually worn longer as tolerated. Red areas are noted prior to and after splint wear. Red areas lasting longer than 15 to t20 minutes indicate that the splint needs adjustment.

Volar Splint with Outrigger

A factory worker has undergone extensor repair of the first two digits of the right hand after suffering a de-gloving injury at work. This person comes into your clinic with an order for a volar splint with outrigger. The splint that is requested would consist of a volar thermoplastic component. The distal two joints of the first and second finger are to remain free, and there will be outrigging over the knuckle of the first two fingers to give it support. These fingers are able to flex but remain supported in extension when not in use. A block to knuckle flexion is placed as specified by the physician as limited flexion allows for reduced excursion of the extensor tendon and allows for healing. The client is trained for independent donning and doffing of the splint as well as a wear schedule. The client is trained in signs of improper fit or placement of the splint. The wear schedule should be gradually increased until the desired time frame is achieved.

Copyright © Mometrix Media. You have been licensed one copy of this document for personal use only. Any other reproduction or redistribution is strictly prohibited. All rights reserved.
This content is provided for test preparation purposes only and does not imply an endorsement by Mometrix of any particular political, scientific, or religious point of view.

Thumb Spica Splint

Thumb spica splints are applied to decrease movement and provide support and comfort to injuries of the scaphoid and lunate bones, first metacarpal fractures, injuries to the ulnar collateral ligament, and positioning for de Quervain tenosynovitis. This splint supports the wrist while isolating the thumb in a slight abducted fashion. The contraindications for this splint include open fractures, injuries involving the neurovascular system, and complicated fractures. Wrist and finger range of motion may begin within a week or two post-surgery or post-injury. Movement is usually prescribed by physicians when they feel mobilization is appropriate. As with all splints, boney prominences should be checked during the use of the splint to prevent pressure areas.

Wrist Cock-Up Splint

The wrist cock-up splint is most commonly used for carpal tunnel syndrome, although it can also be used for fractures, nerve injuries, wrist sprains, tendonitis, ganglion cysts, and arthritis. This splint places the wrist in a neutral or slight extension of the wrist but leaves the fingers free. The benefits of this type of splint is that it is easy to fabricate, cool in temperature to wear, allows firm support of the wrist, and allows for functional use of the fingers and thumb. Customized splints can be easily fabricated. However, there are many prefabricated splints that also work well, save fabrication time and costs, and allow for heated adjustment. Due to the sleek nature of this splint, it also has a good rate of patient compliance. Wrist cock-up splints can be worn day or night as tolerated and recommended or prescribed by the occupational therapist and physician.

Splints for Fractured Elbow

The posterior elbow splint is most commonly used for elbow (olecranon) fractures. This splint is used with soft-tissue injuries of the elbow as well as injuries of the proximal radius and ulna that require immobilization of the wrist and elbow. There are also occasions in which the ordering physician will order the occupational therapist to fabricate a bi-valve cast that can be removed as prescribed for range of motion as well as hygiene. Casts are made of plaster or fiberglass materials. Padding is used inside of the cast to prevent skin breakdown. Although there are some prefabricated splints, custom-made splinting or casting is most common for this type of injury.

Shoulder Immobilizer

The shoulder immobilizer is used on an injured or post-operative shoulder. This device is specifically used after fractures or rotator cuff tears. The shoulder immobilizer is positioned around the shoulder and back, holding the proximal humerus in place. A foam, cylindrical wedge slightly abducts the humerus in abduction. Although this type of immobilizer does not offer as much support as other, more rigid immobilizers, it does allow for some movement for the patient to participate in light daily activities. Shoulder immobilizers can be donned or doffed by the patient. However, training is required, and such a task is often easier with two people. During the early phases of joint mobilization, the immobilizer is taken off for brief periods of time to allow for light exercise. Exercise and time away from the immobilizer are increased based upon doctor and therapist recommendations.

Advantages and Disadvantages of Using Progressive Extension Splints

The progressive extension splint is used to prevent or reverse contractures. This splint usually comes in the form of a metal splint that is hinged and padded for comfort. This splint is worn for several hours with a small amount of pressure applied to the affected joint in the direction opposite the pull of the contracture. For instance, if the joint is contracting into flexion, then extension would be applied to the joint. This device, when it works, greatly reduces contractures. However, there are two main reasons why this splint fails; first, the splint requires perfect alignment with the joint to

Copyright © Mometrix Media. You have been licensed one copy of this document for personal use only. Any other reproduction or redistribution is strictly prohibited. All rights reserved.
This content is provided for test preparation purposes only and does not imply an endorsement by Mometrix of any particular political, scientific, or religious point of view.

prevent pain and skin breakdown. Second, the application of the splint can be so complicated that the primary caregiver is not able to successfully apply the splint.

Training for a Tenodesis Grasp

Quadriplegics at the C5-C6 level will have limited grasp. Allowing for tightening of the hand flexors allows for the ability to automatically partially close the hand when the wrist is extended. This allows for limited grasp for holding items such as a sandwich and a cup. The tenodesis splint is used to assist in the grasp by assisting the index finger and thumb to come closer together to form a grasp as the wrist is extended. The patient is trained, first, in wrist extension. Next, the grasp is used to practice picking up larger objects. As the grasp is achieved through tenodesis, functional objects are used in therapy. The tenodesis grasp is also functional in conjunction shoulder movement for wheelchair propulsion.

Boutonniere Deformity

The Boutonniere deformity is formed by the middle joint of a finger being bent with the distal end of the finger extended. This deformity can happen as a result of a tendon laceration on the back of the finger or from disease processes like rheumatoid arthritis. A splint for Boutonniere's deformity involves a small, wire-based splint that puts pressure on the finger joints in the directions opposite from the deformity. Therefore, the proximal and distal joints of the finger are placed into extension from the volar side of the finger, and the middle finger joint has force placed on it from the dorsal side of the finger. The Boutonniere's deformity decreases the functional use of the hand. Splints slow down the process but do not reverse the damage to tissues.

Anti-Spasticity Splint

The anti-spasticity splint is used to reduced hand and wrist spasticity. The hand is placed into a corrugated finger design using a tennis ball to fabricate the arches of the hand. The fingers are placed in abduction, while the wrist is placed in a neutral position. Modifications to the specifications of the splint can be made based upon the level of spasticity involved with the wrist and hand. The anti-spasticity splint is worn mainly during rest periods to prevent contractures of the wrist and hand due to increased tone. Prolonged stretch is a good tool. However, with spasticity, a limited amount of time may be tolerated using the splint. It is better to get the patient used to the splint by allowing a wearing schedule that includes several short wearing periods rather than one long wearing period.

Cubital Tunnel Syndrome

Cubital tunnel syndrome is one of the more common nerve compression syndromes in the arm. It is caused by increased pressure on the ulnar nerve as it passes through the cubital tunnel of the elbow. The nerve pain associated with bumping this nerve on a surface is what is called the "funny bone." Ulnar nerve syndrome results from prolonged stretching or repeated stretching of the ulnar nerve. There are several ulnar splints. Some splints are placed on the anterior arm, and some are placed on the posterior of the arm. The basic concept is that the elbow is placed in a slight flexion of about 20 degrees to allow relaxation and protection of the ulnar nerve. The splint is worn at all times as tolerated until symptoms subside.

Orthotics

Orthotics is the evaluation, fabrication, and custom fitting of orthopedic braces to control, guide, limit, or immobilize a joint, or limb. Orthotics can assist or restrict movement as well as aid in rehabilitation after the removal of a cast. Orthotics are also used to correct shape and function of a part of the body. For instance, upper extremity orthotics can assist in the extension of elbows to prevent contractures. Common conditions that use orthotics are cerebral palsy, scoliosis, spina

Copyright © Mometrix Media. You have been licensed one copy of this document for personal use only. Any other reproduction or redistribution is strictly prohibited. All rights reserved.
This content is provided for test preparation purposes only and does not imply an endorsement by Mometrix of any particular political, scientific, or religious point of view.

bifida, traumatic brain injury, multiple sclerosis, and sports injuries. Occupational therapists fabricate some orthotics as well as rely on basic knowledge to select prefabricated orthotics for the upper body. In some cases, custom-made orthotics are necessary. Orthotists are often consulted to determine whether custom-made or prefabricated orthotics are recommended.

Enabling Participation with Durable Medical Equipment

Measuring for Seating Positioning Systems for Power Mobility

The following measurements are taken when measuring for a power mobility seating system: hip width, widest point across lower extremities, chest width, heel to knee length, coccyx to posterior knee length, elbow to coccyx length, shoulder height, head height, hip width, widest point of chest, and foot to posterior knee length. Things to consider when ordering a powerchair are the following: The chair should last at least 5 years. Anticipate any changes in health condition that may necessitate surgery and a subsequent change in seating options. Anticipate weight gain or loss based upon medical status. Discuss with the patient previous medical history of skin breakdown. If much change is expected over the use of the new powerchair, then a chair that allows for expansion or reduction of seating components may be necessary.

Methodology Behind a Mat Assessment for Seating

A mat assessment is important as it helps determine seating angles and support surfaces necessary for the client. The mat assessment is done both sitting and supine. In supine, the pelvis is examined to determine if it can achieve a neutral position. Spine symmetry as well as pelvic tilt (posterior or anterior tilt) is examined to determine if the pelvis can achieve a neutral position. Observations regarding if there is a pelvic obliquity (pelvic rotation) are also important. In sitting, the position of the head and neck to the trunk is observed. Control of the trunk while sitting supported and unsupported determines the need for lateral supports on the chair. Using the assessment of these items, the proper seat-to-back angle can be recommended.

Choosing Between Prefabricated Seating System or Custom-Made Seating System

Therapists often question whether to use custom or off-the-shelf seating systems for a client. There are a couple of simple rules to follow to determine whether to recommend one seating system over the other. Clients who have more symmetrical pelvic measurements may need less custom seating. Those who have pelvic and/or spinal deformities may require custom-built seating. The same is true for spinal deformities. Some minor spinal deformities may require only off-the-shelf seating systems, whereas extreme spinal deformities may require custom seating. Many off-the-shelf seating systems are now adjustable and allow for greater flexibility depending upon the client's needs. The occupational therapist should always collaborate with a representative from a good medical supply company to determine products available for a particular patient.

Wedges to Position Torso in a Wheelchair to Compensate for Lateral Scoliosis

Lateral positioning is usually accomplished through wedges that are foam or gel filled. Wedges come in different lengths and densities depending upon the client's measurements. Wedges are meant to correct lateral tilt of the torso toward one direct while sitting in a wheelchair. The mat evaluation determines where best to place the wedge. Wedges attach to the canes (the upright posts of the seat back). A wedge that is placed on the right side will compensate for the patient who tilts toward the right side and vice versa. If the mat evaluation reveals that the patient has poor control of both right and left sitting balance, then one wedge may be placed in a higher position on one side, and another wedge may be placed in a lower position on the opposite side.

Copyright © Mometrix Media. You have been licensed one copy of this document for personal use only. Any other reproduction or redistribution is strictly prohibited. All rights reserved.
This content is provided for test preparation purposes only and does not imply an endorsement by Mometrix of any particular political, scientific, or religious point of view.

Using Tilt or Recline in a Power Wheelchair

Reclining a wheelchair opens the seat-to-back angle and is used in combination with elevating the leg rests. Reclining is used to redistribute pressure from the hips and buttock areas for comfort, for sitting tolerance, and to reduce the risk of skin breakdown. Contraindications for reclining are spasticity, some head injuries, and muscle diseases that have associated spasticity. Tilt is used to also reduce the risk of pressure sores and for comfort. Tilt can be used to elicit extensor tone. Often, tilt is used when range of motion prohibits either hip extension or hip flexion due to tight musculature. However, in a tilt position, it will be harder for a patient to work at a table. Some patients may experience bladder emptying problems also. Finally, the ability to have a chair tilt and recline is a good option for patients who become agitated, uncomfortable, or hurt when staying in one position for long periods of time.

Selecting a Seating Surface

Seating surfaces vary from foam to gel to air (among the basic components). Choosing among seating surfaces depends upon the patient's medical condition as well as past medical history. Patients who use a wheelchair for infrequent outings and have no history of skin breakdown benefit from a foam surface. Patients who sit for longer periods of time may benefit from a gel surface. Those patients who have a history of skin breakdowns but currently are breakdown free should be placed on a gel surface. However, those patients with active skin breakdown should be placed on an air surface. There are also cushions that combine different surfaces. One such cushion has air cells in the center with gel padding on the perimeter of the cushion. This cushion would be used for someone who has a very localized wound toward the coccyx area.

Medicare Criteria for Power Mobility

The first criteria for a powerchair is a face-to-face exam by a physician as well as a referral for a therapy evaluation for the need of a powerchair. The criteria for a powerchair consists of the inability of a client to push a manual wheelchair due to illness or injury. The client has to be cognitively able to maneuver a chair with or without adaptations. Additionally, the client must have the ability to safely transfer to and from the powerchair safely. Operation of the chair within the home is considered only. A power wheelchair offers a tight turning radius. However, when medical need does not indicate specialized power mobility, a scooter may be sufficient. Scooters are larger and often more difficult to maneuver in the home. Therefore, powerchairs are more frequently recommended.

Low- and High-Tech Devices

Low-tech devices involve little or no technology. High-tech devices usually involve technology such as computing devices. These devices aid forms of communication such as writing, reading, and speaking. Low- and high-tech devices are used across the life span from school-age children with cerebral palsy to adults with stroke. Communication devices can be used in the job setting also (provided essential functions of the job can be completed). As computers become smaller and quicker, the processing and speech generated from high-tech devices become more natural and truer to human speech. Higher-tech devices are often not covered with traditional insurance and, instead, are provided through state programs that offer funds for certain disabilities.

Choosing an Assistive Device to Recommend for a Client

When choosing an assistive device, there are many considerations to consider. First, one must consider the purpose of what the assistive technology will be used for as well as the setting in which it will be used. Second, the cognitive level of the person should be considered. For instance, some clients may benefit from many choices available on the communication board, and some may

Copyright © Mometrix Media. You have been licensed one copy of this document for personal use only. Any other reproduction or redistribution is strictly prohibited. All rights reserved.
This content is provided for test preparation purposes only and does not imply an endorsement by Mometrix of any particular political, scientific, or religious point of view.

benefit from fewer choices. It is also important, especially with more expensive equipment, to find something that is adaptable to the future as well as something that is beneficial for the present. Finally, it is imperative to make sure that the device is age appropriate to avoid stigmatizing the user. The ultimate goal is to increase the quality of life for the client as well as make him or her more independent.

OT's Role in Use of Low- and High-Tech Devices

School Settings

In a school setting, the occupational therapist's (OT's) role is to make sure the student is able to perform the tasks necessary to learn. Low-tech devices take the form of built-up writing devices, assistive devices used to help punch the keys of a computer, magnifying glasses for reading, as well as aids used to dress and toilet at school. The OT relies on the teacher to describe the expectations and difficulties the student is experiencing. Low-tech communication boards involve a picture and the cognitive ability for the child to understand the symbolism and point to the correct picture representation. Higher-tech devices such as communication boards that mount on wheelchairs and portable communication boards are ordered based upon recommendations from the OT evaluation and speech therapy evaluation. Collaboration with the family and teachers define which communication board is appropriate for the student.

Communication

Occupational therapists (OTs) are instrumental in providing the tools necessary to meet the demands of the task. Occupational therapists have the skills necessary to assess clients and provide assistive technology devices. Especially important is to assess the client's performance, abilities, preferences, environmental context, and barriers to the technology device features. The OT also collaborates with educators, assistive technology providers, manufacturers, and the client and family. It is the responsibility of the OT to be familiar with available technology and have a basic working knowledge on how to use the devices. OTs must also understand how devices interface with each other. For instance, some communication devices mount on the power mobility device. It is best to know the make and model of the mobility device that the communication device will be attached to recommend the proper position of the device.

Work Environment

Within the work environment, there is opportunity for both low- and high-tech devices. An occupational therapist's (OT's) assessment in the clinic or at the client's work environment will reveal areas needing ergonomic improvements. Devices such as ergonomic keyboards are designed to minimize strain on the upper body, shoulders, and back. Screen readers are high-tech devices that use software to read print. These devices are used mainly by blind clients. Voice recognition software is used for those individuals who need assistance to type due to disease, limb loss, or arthritis. Screen magnifiers make text larger for low vision employees and is another example of a low-tech device. Ergonomic chairs offer additional adjustments that most office chairs do not offer and offer a good option for those individuals with chronic back pain. There are endless devices that the OT can use to creatively shape the environment of the patient.

Caregiver's Role in Assisting Client to Use Low- and High-Tech Devices

A client who requires assistive technology in the school, work, or home setting will often need to practice and become efficient with the equipment. The therapist only has limited time within the work, therapy, and school setting to work with the client. A home program designed to become acquainted with the assistive device is important to be successful in the actual usage environment. Settings for many low- and high- tech devices can be modified based upon feedback from the client and family. Additional support in adjusting the programming of a device is often referred to the

Copyright © Mometrix Media. You have been licensed one copy of this document for personal use only. Any other reproduction or redistribution is strictly prohibited. All rights reserved.
This content is provided for test preparation purposes only and does not imply an endorsement by Mometrix of any particular political, scientific, or religious point of view.

vendor for the device as special software is many times required to reprogram features on the device. The OT also offers ongoing support should any issues arise with the device.

Adaptive Keyboards for Students with Cerebral Palsy and Limited Hand Range of Motion

The first step toward assessing any limitations is to observe the student typing. In a school setting the goal of therapy would not be to correct any hand limitations but to find an adaptive keyboard that would allow this student to type and complete assignments. There are various keyboards to consider. It the problem was limited motor accuracy and control, an expanded keyboard that has larger keys may provide the correct adaptation to allow this student to complete work. However, if the evaluation reveals that the main problem is limited range of motion, then a miniature keyboard may allow for better accuracy. There is also the availability of a light touch keyboard for people with limited hand strength. In some cases, speech recognition software may provide an alternative when adaptations have failed.

Suggestions for Student Who Sustained Burns and Can't Type or Take Notes in School

A client who was in a house fire and sustained second- and third-degree burns over 60% of the body (arms, hands, chest, and legs) expresses to you that he or she may have to drop out of college because he or she cannot use his or her hands to type papers or take notes. The burned hand may take many months to heal and regain function. However, in the interim, there are several things to do that will assist the client to function in a college environment. First, there are several software programs available for purchase that allow for voice recognition. While therapy progresses and, hopefully, function is restored, this is a good alternative. Second, there are several pieces of adaptive equipment that will fit into a universal cuff or wrap around the hand and allow for typing using a stylus. Incorporate practicing typing into the therapy session. Typing can increase finger range of motion as well as strength. Finally, in the absence of being able to take notes during class, suggest recording lectures. If lectures cannot be recorded, the client may need to ask others to take notes.

Mobility Options for a Grocery Store

Mobility options for a grocery store can take the form of devices brought by the client or devices available at the store. Both have advantages and disadvantages. The client can bring devices such as a cane, walker, or four-wheeled rollator. The cane (a single point or a multi-point cane) requires the use of balance while reaching for objects in the store. A rollator or walker uses both hands to maneuver. Therefore, with less balance and two hands being occupied with mobility, it is even harder to reach for objects on shelves. A power chair or scooter is another option for those who are able to stand to reach objects safely but cannot walk the distances required in a store. When safety is questionable, it is better to have a caregiver, family member, or friend assist in grocery shopping.

Vehicle Adaptations

Vehicle adaptations refer to additions made to the car to assist in driving, stowage, and access. Driving adaptations most commonly come in the form of knobs added to the steering wheel for maneuvering the vehicle. Accelerator adaptations for the foot or to use by hand can be other adaptations. There are even remote-control devices to drive a car. Stowage refers to adding a lift or above-roof storage case to carry wheelchairs and power mobility. Devices for access usually involve adaptations to the vehicle so that the client can drive a powerchair into the car or van and either drive from the wheelchair level or be placed in the passenger's side of the van. In some cases, access involves lowering the floor of the van to accommodate a powerchair with an occupant in the chair.

Copyright © Mometrix Media. You have been licensed one copy of this document for personal use only. Any other reproduction or redistribution is strictly prohibited. All rights reserved.
This content is provided for test preparation purposes only and does not imply an endorsement by Mometrix of any particular political, scientific, or religious point of view.

Steering Wheel Adaptations

There are several devices available to adapt the steering wheel to limited hand motion. These accommodations are most commonly used by clients with quadriplegia, arthritis, stroke, or any disease process that limits the hand and shoulder motion necessary to operate a steering wheel. These devices mount onto the steering wheel and allow for turning the wheel via things such as a steering glove, steering balls, and steering tetra grip. These devices allow for the driver to have complete control of the vehicle with only one hand. Sometimes the size of the steering wheel has to be reduced in size, such as when the driver is driving from a wheelchair. Finally, there are infrared steering devices that can allow for the same hand that is steering to operate the secondary controls.

Options for Making Lifting Wheelchairs Easier

A daughter wishes to take her elderly mother to dinner but complains that each time she has taken her mother, her hands hurt from lifting the wheelchair into the car. Lifting a standard wheelchair is difficult as they can weigh close to 40 pounds. Additionally, they are big and bulky and sometimes do not fit in smaller vehicles. A lightweight wheelchair is a few pounds lighter and many times can be folded and placed into the backseat or trunk of a car. The lightest weight option for the daughter of this patient would be a travel wheelchair. These chairs are not only very lightweight (weighing under 20 pounds) but can be folded from the center and will take up less of footprint in a vehicle. This is the best option to fit in economy and compact sized vehicles. The occupational therapist is involved in training the family and patient in car transfers and proper body mechanics during transfers.

Options for Patients Who Do Not Have Access to a Car

Many individuals do not have a car or someone to transport them. In these instances, public transportation can often fill the need. Most public transportation systems have disability services in the form of a special van that is wheelchair accessible or a cab service. There are often private services that can offer transportation to those qualified clients. A social worker is able to connect qualified clients with the appropriate service and assist in completing necessary paperwork. Most transportation services also need the signed authorization of a doctor. The disadvantage to such services is that they are sometimes late, often make several stops to pick up other clients, and take an extended period of time to arrive at a destination.

Treatment Performed in Driver Rehabilitation Department

The occupational therapist in the field of driver rehabilitation will often have a Certified Driver Rehabilitation Specialist certification. Access to simulators are important to evaluate and treat the patient who wants to return to driving. Simulators can simulate any number of situations to test for visual field deficits, neglect of one side, safety awareness, and motor control of the steering wheel, pedals, and knobs. On-the-road training involves training to safely operate a vehicle with and without adaptations. This is the stage during which recommendations for adaptations are made. In some instances, new vehicles with specified parameters are purchased for or by the patient to be adapted to prescribed needs. Driver rehabilitation can be an extended process that requires patience from all involved.

Certified Driver Rehabilitation Specialist Certification Requirements

The occupational therapist who wants to apply for the Certified Driver Rehabilitation Specialist exam must have 1,664 hours of experience providing direct driver rehabilitation. It is suggested to spend time with those who already have the certification. Read as much as possible and attend as many conferences and continuing education classes as possible. There are also web sources for online classes, webinars, and reading materials that are helpful to prepare for the exam. The

Copyright © Mometrix Media. You have been licensed one copy of this document for personal use only. Any other reproduction or redistribution is strictly prohibited. All rights reserved.
This content is provided for test preparation purposes only and does not imply an endorsement by Mometrix of any particular political, scientific, or religious point of view.

Association for Driver Rehabilitation Specialists is also a good organization to join as they are the premier organization for this field and offer numerous resources to their members. Finally, the exam preparation manual offers tips and practice questions to study for the exam.

Role of Maintenance on Reliability and Longevity of Devices

A device (high or low tech) is only as good as its reliability. For a device to remain consistent, it must regularly be maintained. This is why maintenance should be part of patient education upon the client's receiving a new piece of equipment. Those devices with batteries, such as patient lifts and power wheelchairs, need to be charged on a regular basis to maintain the health of the battery. Manual wheelchairs need to be cleaned on a regular basis for the wheels to smoothly role. Due to being made of partially biodegradable materials, slings for lifts have an expiration date and need to be replaced as indicated. It is important for instructions to be read by caregivers also as patients with medical and/or cognitive issues sometimes do not readily remember instructions.

Sanitizing Durable Medical Equipment Between Patients

There are some pieces of medical equipment that cannot be used between patients. Items such as bedside commodes, tub benches, and shower chairs can be used by only one person. Items such as wheelchairs, lifts, and dressing aids can be used by more than one person as long as they are sanitized between different patients. The quickest and most efficient way to sanitize a piece of equipment is to spray it with a hospital-grade solution such as Wexide. The item should soak in the solution for 10 minutes prior to drying. A second choice for disinfection is to wipe down the device with a disinfectant wipe. Again, leave the solution on the item for 10 minutes prior to drying. In some instances, if the item has visible dirt, it will need to be hand washed prior to disinfecting.

Relationship Between Device Complexity and Patient Compliance

In considering what device to order a patient, there are many factors to consider. One of the most important factors is whether or not the patient will actually use the device purchased. For any category of adaptive devices there are numerous choices to consider. However, it is not always wise to get the device that has all of the "bells and whistles." Although fancy devices may seem appealing to an occupational therapist, they are often difficult for patients and family members to comprehend. Thus, the device is not used. It is much preferred to order simpler devices that may not be as fancy but may be better suited to the patient and family. An assessment of cognition as well as personal history will often lead to a clear understanding of the level of complexity of the assistive device.

Home Evaluation for Patient Receiving Hip Replacement Surgery

The two things that you will need to look for are fall risks in the home and medical equipment that will need to be ordered. Hazards in the home may consist of throw rugs, stairways, steps to entrances, uneven walkways, and seating surfaces that are too low (considering hip precaution of not bending hip over ninety degrees). Medical equipment that will need to be considered is an elevated toilet seat, a bench for the tub or shower (transfer bench for tub), elevating the height of couches and chairs with risers, and ramps if the patient is wheelchair bound. Hip precautions last only a few months but prevent hip dislocation and subsequent falls. All activities need to be conducted within the tolerance of pain and no further.

Importance of Patient Perception and Appearance with Relation to Adaptive Equipment

One of the most important factors influencing patients' use of equipment is their perception of themselves using the equipment. If the equipment is sleek and attractive to the patient, there is a higher chance of compliance with usage. This is why it is important to involve the patient in the

Copyright © Mometrix Media. You have been licensed one copy of this document for personal use only. Any other reproduction or redistribution is strictly prohibited. All rights reserved.
This content is provided for test preparation purposes only and does not imply an endorsement by Mometrix of any particular political, scientific, or religious point of view.

selection process. In some cases, there will need to be a compromise. For example, if a patient prefers one model wheelchair over another, then a comparison of features needs to take place. It may be necessary to give up some features in the therapist's preferred chair for the patient to agree and use the device. In the instance in which it is important for the patient to have a particular feature, the therapist should explain the advantages and offer aesthetic alternatives that the patient will agree to as a tradeoff for added function.

Training Methods for Different Learning Styles

The three basic learning styles are auditory, visual, and tactile. The auditory learning client prefers listening to instructions as the primary method of learning. The visual client prefers seeing visualizations such as pictures, drawings, and schematics to learn. This type of learner will like videos such as those found on YouTube to learn how to use a piece of adaptive equipment. Finally, the tactile learner prefers to actually practice using the device rather than viewing films or solely listening to explanations. The preferred method for teaching the use of adaptive equipment for most therapists is a combination of tactile and auditory styles. It is mainly through practice and repetitions that clients are best able to learn to perform needed tasks to use adaptive equipment.

Educating Staff on DME

As new products become available, there needs to be a method to incorporate durable medical equipment (DME) education in the staff education plan. Although the DME supplier is the ultimate expert in product information, the occupational therapist should have a good working knowledge of available DME. Staff education is often achieved through vendor in-services or vendor continuing education. The advantage of the in-service format is that it can be done in the therapy clinic. This method is usually limited in time as it occurs prior to or after treatment times or during lunch. The continuing education course is usually offered off site and brings in subject matter experts to discuss the topic. This type of education can last several hours. In-services that offer labs are best as they allow for a hands-on approach.

Training Methods for Sliding Tub Bench

The sliding tub bench is a good example of a product that needs a combination of learning styles. The auditory and tactile styles of learning can be incorporated into training on most durable medical equipment (DME). Practice is necessary for therapists also. The learning curve is quick but, nonetheless, will often reveal new methods of use of the equipment. Repetitive practice on more complex DME allows for thorough understanding and a better chance to be able to adequately teach patients and family members. In using the tactile method of teaching, it is often best to show an example of how the medical equipment is used prior to having the patient and family practice with the item.

Guidelines, Standards, and Legislation for Environmental Modifications

ADA Compliant

The Americans for Disabilities Act (ADA) states that buildings, structures, site improvements, and pedestrian routes must maintain access for people with disabilities. Specifically, facilities must be wheelchair accessible. Areas such as doorways, sidewalks, theater seating, and bathrooms require electronic doorways, ramps, and other appropriate accommodations for people with disabilities. There are standards available for new buildings as well as older buildings needing to remodel to comply with ADA standards. Dimensions are standardized for egresses, parking spaces, passenger loading zones, stairways, drinking fountains, kitchens, bathrooms, amusement areas, as well as all

Copyright © Mometrix Media. You have been licensed one copy of this document for personal use only. Any other reproduction or redistribution is strictly prohibited. All rights reserved.
This content is provided for test preparation purposes only and does not imply an endorsement by Mometrix of any particular political, scientific, or religious point of view.

public areas. Fines are assessed for noncompliance to standards. ADA standards are important for therapists to know (based upon the settings in which they practice) as many times clients are returning home after a hospitalization and face new challenges due to a new disability. ADA standards allow therapists to recommend home improvements so that clients can access all areas of their homes.

Ergonomics

Ergonomics is the study of how work is accomplished using the most efficient means possible. Efficiency, with relation to ergonomics, is reducing the strength required to perform physical effort, reducing the number of steps to complete a task, or making instructions simpler to reduce the amount of training needed. Efficiency not only has to do with effort but also makes things safer. Ergonomic design can also reduce the chances of repetitive strain injuries (especially in the hand). By reducing repetition, strain injuries such as carpal tunnel, cubital tunnel, and tenosynovitis can be reduced. Ergonomics also increases worker productivity and attendance as fewer injuries occur requiring time away from work. Occupational therapists can print any number of informational pages from numerous web pages on the Internet.

Universal Design

Universal design is the design and creation of an environment that can be accessed, understood, and used by people of all ages and disabilities. By considering the diverse needs and abilities of all people throughout the design process, universal design creates products, services, and environments that meet peoples' needs. Certain standards dictate the width of doorways, countertop heights, space allowed for the turning radius of a wheelchair, grade required for ramps, height for toilets, as well as requirements for grab bars (to name a few). Universal design incorporates professions such as occupational therapists, architects, and contractors to complete the building or remodeling process. There are also several certifications that incorporate universal design as a central concept in redesigning the home for the elderly, sick, and handicapped.

Certification Programs and Continuing Education for Universal Design

There are several universal design certifications available for occupational therapists (OTs). The Certified Aging in Place Specialist (CAPS) is one such certification that focuses on the technical aspects, business management, and customer service skills for modifications. Courses taken in this certification are marketing and communication, design concepts for livable homes and aging in place, and detailed solutions for livable homes and aging in place. The Certified Home Assessment and Modification Professional (CHAMPS) trains the OT to assess, contract, communicate with insurance companies, and oversee construction of modifications. The American Occupational Therapy Association also has a continuing education certification that focuses on home modifications. This course can be completed online. Finally, the American Society on Aging offers an online program on housing design, accessibility, and technology. These are a few of the several programs available for OTs.

Assessing Universal Design in the Home

Occupational therapists (OTs) are able to obtain any number of certifications in universal design and ergonomics. This knowledge base is aimed at assessing the individual in his or her home, work space, school, or anywhere the individual spends a majority of the day or night. Issues such as narrow doorways, countertops that are too high, accessible entrances to homes and buildings, redesigning the bathroom for a roll-in shower and elevated commode, grab bars, ramps, stair lifts, and automation within the home are examples of universal design changes considered by the OT. Collaboration is made with the patient to determine funds available and what can be accomplished

Copyright © Mometrix Media. You have been licensed one copy of this document for personal use only. Any other reproduction or redistribution is strictly prohibited. All rights reserved.
This content is provided for test preparation purposes only and does not imply an endorsement by Mometrix of any particular political, scientific, or religious point of view.

with those funds. The OT also assists in making sure changes to the home are made within specified guidelines.

Implementing Universal Design in the Home

Occupational therapists (OTs) can assist in more than just the evaluation. OTs provide evaluations to contractors so they are able to determine home specification for remodeling. The OT can also, with some certifications, be the lead in arranging contract work as well as project timelines. Periodically, the OT will visit the construction site to ensure construction is within the paraments agreed upon. Upon conclusion, the OT trains the patient and family in mobility in the newly renovated space, transfers, and features incorporated into the design to make the patient more independent. New items such as transfer shower wheelchairs, handheld showers, and grab bars are often added once construction is complete.

Rules for Universal Design in Public Places of Business

The universal design for public places involves things such as installing standard electrical receptacles higher than usual so they can be reached by everyone, selecting wider doors, making flat entrances, adding ramped entrances, replacing handles on doorways with loop handles, making sure all cabinets and storage spaces are within reach of all. In the workplace universal design means wide-open spaces so that all people can more easily reach and access shelves and storage areas. Occupational therapists not only consult and are active in the construction phase of universal design for the home but are also active in universal design for the business. The Americans with Disabilities Act states specific laws for accessing public places that must be adhered to during the planning and construction phases.

Reasonable Accommodation

A company is required to modify its work environment to meet the needs of a returning injured worker as long as the accommodation does not entail undue hardship to the company (pertaining to companies with 15+ employees). Reasonable accommodation is not specifically defined and remains to be determined by the company. For instance, a secretary who has had carpal tunnel surgery may need a special ergonomic keyboard and mouse, a computer table that adjusts to an ergonomic height, and an adjustable-height monitor. This accommodation would likely be considered reasonable considering the cost would be low. However, if the same client were to request all handles on the facility's doorknobs be fitted with ergonomic handles, this would be considered unreasonable. The cost to replace all doorknob handles would outweigh the benefit provided to one employee.

Procedure for Reasonable Accommodations in the Work Environment

An employee can request accommodations, and the employer must respond to the request within 30 business days from the date the request was made. Medical records, such as an occupational therapist (OT) evaluation may be requested. If an evaluation has not been completed, then the company may request the primary physician order an OT evaluation. Once the evaluation is complete, the report can be sent to the employer. The employer should make every effort to complete the recommended work within as short of a period as possible. If the employee feels reasonable accommodations are not being made in a timely fashion, the Equal Employment Opportunity office can be contacted. The OT can assist the employee and employer by informing both of the Americans with Disabilities act (ADA) specifications for ramps, turning radius for wheelchairs, bathroom specifications, and ergonomic improvements for the employee at his or her workstation.

Copyright © Mometrix Media. You have been licensed one copy of this document for personal use only. Any other reproduction or redistribution is strictly prohibited. All rights reserved.
This content is provided for test preparation purposes only and does not imply an endorsement by Mometrix of any particular political, scientific, or religious point of view.

Ergonomic Factors for Desk Job for Client with Lumbar Back Pain

A desk job means the client spends many hours daily sitting performing his or her job. This allows for stiff joints, increased pain, and possible blood clots. Ergonomics center on a proper seating position in which the arms are at a 90-degree bend. Hands must be level with the keyboard, and the computer screen should be at eye level with no bend at the neck. All items on the desk should be at the height between the shoulder and waist level. When sitting, hips and knees should be at 90 degrees. Also, of importance is the fact that every hour of sitting should be broken up with 5 minutes of standing or walking to prevent blood clots.

Identifying and Remediating Contributing Factors to Carpal Tunnel in Client's Workplace

A client who is a cashier at a grocery store comes into your clinic post carpal tunnel surgery. Carpal tunnel is prevalent among cashiers. The occupational therapist can assist the client not only physically but also by recommending the following preventative steps. First, try a softer touch. Many times, individuals are so familiar with a task that they tend to overdo actions, for instance, depressing keys much harder than necessary on a keyboard. This causes tension as well as pain and can contribute to overuse. Second, break for a few minutes every hour to allow for some recovery from the repetitive motion of typing. When resting, it is a good idea to perform upper-body stretches to keep limber. Next, wear a brace when sleeping to avoid overstretching of tissues. Finally, be mindful of posture.

Ramp Evaluation for a Home Setting

To measure for a ramp, therapists first add the total height of the steps. For instance, if there are four steps to a porch and each step is 4 inches tall, the total height will be 16 inches. Therefore, the ramp will need to cover 16 inches of total height. The ADA standard for length is 1:12. For every inch of height there must be 1 foot of ramp. So, for 16 inches of height, the ramp will need to extend 192 inches or 16 feet. A ramp that is longer than 6 inches should have handrails. Some ramps, depending upon available space, may need to curve. It is also important to add a non-skid surface to the ramp as many metal ramps are slick. Smaller ramps that cover thresholds are often made of rubber and can be cut to fit doorways.

Factors in Implementation of Home Modifications

There are several factors that can affect the home modification process. Funding is a factor that will ultimately determine whether all, some, or none of the modifications are possible to complete. Once the evaluation process is complete, a contractor determines the cost of modifications. Factors influencing cost are materials, extent of work to be completed (older homes may require extensive plumbing work), and time to complete. It is always better for the client to agree to a few modifications done well and with top-grade materials than agreeing to extensive modifications using cheap materials and done poorly. Additionally, some communities require permits prior to starting work. This can be a lengthy and frustrating process. The occupational therapist can expedite the process by acting as a liaison among all involved parties.

Resources for Locating DME for Patient's Home

The age of therapists carrying stacks of catalogues in their cars to identify sources of durable medical equipment (DME) are long gone. Due to the fact that most home health occupational therapists (OTs) are given laptops or tablets allows clinicians the ability to look up DME companies in a matter of seconds. Companies such as Performance Medical, Alimed, and North Coast medical offer extensive online catalogues available for referencing and ordering. Also, over time, therapists should learn the representatives name from companies such as Quickie, Pride Mobility, Hill-Rom,

Copyright © Mometrix Media. You have been licensed one copy of this document for personal use only. Any other reproduction or redistribution is strictly prohibited. All rights reserved.
This content is provided for test preparation purposes only and does not imply an endorsement by Mometrix of any particular political, scientific, or religious point of view.

and other notable providers of larger DME. The OT involved in modifications will also know contract companies that are licensed to provide universal design modifications to the home. This is an endless task as sources for DME are always changing. One method to keep up with this fast-changing industry is continuing education seminars.

Safety Concerns When Performing Home Evaluation in Client's Bathroom

The bathroom is the easiest place to fall within a home. This happens because of slippery floors, slippery feet, throw rugs, and improper transfer technique. It is important to assess for the need of a transfer shower chair or a transfer tub bench. Often, it is necessary to recommend grab bars for areas requiring holding onto a surface to avoid slippage. A handheld shower alleviates the need to stand during bathing as the hose is long enough to sit while showering. The toilet area also needs to be assessed for raised toilet seats and grab bars. Finally, wheelchair-bound clients need to have access to countertop space to reach toiletries.

Adapting a Tub to Allow for Bathing After Hip Surgery

One of the precautions of hip surgery is not bending the hip joint greater than 90 degrees. To get inside the tub, this person's hip precautions would be violated. Additionally, this person will be at a risk for falls for the next several months as he or she recovers from hip surgery. It is important to eliminate this fall risk by providing adaptive equipment. A transfer tub bench extends over the side of the tub and into the tub. With the connection of a handheld shower, the tub bench would be the safest option for this client. Care should be given to the fact that some tubs are sunken as well as garden style. This poses an extra challenge as the legs to the tub bench need to be long enough to extend into the tub.

Working with Apartment Complex to Make Modifications for Client

You perform a home evaluation on a client who lives in an apartment. One of your recommendations is to place grab bars in the bathroom. Your client responds by saying that the apartment complex has previously not agreed to modifications in the bathroom. Your first responsibility is to your client. That being said, modifications can take place (even as simple as installing grab bars) only with the apartment's approval. Many apartment complexes will allow the installation of grab bars. Maintenance staff are usually the ones to install grab bars. In this case, you should make a trip to the manager's office and plead your case with the manager. Explain the risk of falls and injuries in the bathroom without grab bars (one-third of seniors fall each year in the bathroom). Then explain how grab bars prevent falls. Explain that grab bars are removeable once the apartment is vacated. Many times, this logic will seem reasonable to a manager, and he or she will agree to allow the grab bars to be installed.

Kitchen Adaptations for Clients with Total Hip Arthroplasty

A patient with a total hip arthroplasty will have the standard hip precautions. Therefore, items in the kitchen will have to be evaluated for correct height as well as weight. A general rule of thumb is not to have any cooking objects stored above shoulder level or below waist level. Depending upon the surgeon, there will most likely be a weight restriction for carrying objects such as groceries, pots or pans of food, and so on. It is also imperative to teach functional mobility with a walker for things such as retrieving food from the refrigerator, microwave oven, stove, and oven. A functional task such as meal preparation allows the therapist to observe the client maneuvering in a kitchen as well as problem-solving any obstacles that may arise. Finally, countertop space should be optimized to allow for sliding plates or bowls to nearby tables.

Copyright © Mometrix Media. You have been licensed one copy of this document for personal use only. Any other reproduction or redistribution is strictly prohibited. All rights reserved.
This content is provided for test preparation purposes only and does not imply an endorsement by Mometrix of any particular political, scientific, or religious point of view.

Recommendations to Help Newly Wheelchair Bound Patient in the Kitchen

A home health patient who is newly wheelchair bound is assessed by an occupational therapist. Upon completion of the assessment, one of the findings is that the patient cannot reach the kitchen sink or items in the upper cabinets. Additionally, this patient cannot enter the pantry due to the doorway being too narrow. The first recommendation would be to widen the door to the pantry. Second, many sinks have cabinet space under them. By eliminating the cabinet space and creating an opening under the sink, this patient will be able to roll under the sink with the wheelchair and perform necessary tasks. It is not always feasible to remodel a whole kitchen. When this is not possible, train the client to place objects that are most used in lower, reachable cabinets and those less-often-used items in higher cabinets. Some items such as frequently used dishes can even be left on the countertop. In many cases, the patient does not have funds available to implement all recommendation. In this event, a discussion between the patient and therapist should focus on prioritizing patient needs.

Modifications for Safe Transfer on or off the Bed

There are many circumstances that can influence the ability to transfer safely to and from a bed. Assuming that the bed is the correct height and the mattress is not too soft, the next issue that needs to be examined is whether or not there is something that can be used to stabilize the patient while sitting on the edge of the bed to transfer. For some people, a walker in front of the bed provides enough stability. However, for other people, it is necessary to use a bed rail. There are several brands of bed rails that can be used with a regular bed. Most rails involve tucking part of the rail between the mattress and box springs for stability. There should also be some form of legs that extend from the bed rail to the floor. This provides the necessary support to hold onto and to bear weight while performing sit to stand as well as transfers.

Implementing Environmental Modifications in School Settings for Children with ADHD

Students with attention deficit hyperactivity disorder (ADHD) have a difficult time sitting still, concentrating, and listening to others. The occupational therapist can assist in modifying the classroom environment for the student by making a few recommendations. First, eliminate distractions. This may mean to locate the student away from doors, windows, and anything that could pose a distraction. Second, prevent chattering and disrupting behavior by setting rules for the classroom and not wavering from them. Impulsivity can be reduced by also setting classroom rules and rewarding good behavior. Fidgeting can be reduced by incorporating physical movement into the lesson plans so that excess energy can be burned off. Finally, keep instructions and explanations brief, and break down complex tasks into manageable subtasks.

Copyright © Mometrix Media. You have been licensed one copy of this document for personal use only. Any other reproduction or redistribution is strictly prohibited. All rights reserved.
This content is provided for test preparation purposes only and does not imply an endorsement by Mometrix of any particular political, scientific, or religious point of view.

Upholding Professional Standards and Responsibilities

Employing Evidence-Based Strategies

Online Medical Reference Search Engines for Scholarly Research

There are endless medical search engines online. However, there are a few that are considered basic due to their vast databases, interfaces with other search engines, and ease of use. PubMed is one of the leading search engines. This search engine is free and contains more than 25 million records. PubMed also interconnects with Medline. Ovid and ProQuest are other good sources that are relatively easy to use and interface with other databases. OT Seeker and OT Search are databases specific to occupational therapy (OT) that searches journal articles from OT publications. Finally, Google Scholar is a database that has a vast web of connected resources and is easy to search. It is always wise to use more than one database when doing research.

OT Professional Organizations That Offer Scholarly Articles Online

The American Occupational Therapy Association (AOTA) is a good source for research. Most occupational therapists (OTs) belong to this organization and would, therefore, have access to their articles. Information and interest sections on most areas of OT can be found through AOTA online. Additionally, there are state organizations offering online resources also. The World Wide Web connects people from all countries. Just as the United States has a professional organization for OTs, so too do most countries. Perhaps some of the best resources for information come from the Canadian Occupational Therapy Association and the Australian Occupational Therapy Association. The reference section of articles is also a good place to find related articles and topics. Finally, do not forget to look in local and university libraries.

Common Sections in Scholarly Articles

A scholarly article is usually divided into standard sections. Those sections are literature review, research methods, results, discussions and conclusions, and references. The first few paragraphs of a journal article introduce the topic. The hypothesis or thesis is stated that indicates the purpose of the research. The research methods section describes procedures and methods that were used to carry out the research. The discussion and conclusion sections summarize what the results of the research might mean to the field, how the research addresses the original hypothesis, weaknesses of the study, and areas for future research. The reference section lists, in alphabetical order, the authors cited in the body of the work. Appendices often have graphs, photos, or other content referred to in the body of the study.

CQI

Continuous quality improvement (CQI) is a management philosophy that organizations use to reduce waste, increase efficiency, and increase internal (employee) and external (patient) satisfaction. This is an ongoing process. The underlying concept behind CQI is when problems arise, they are a result of poor work design, unclear instructions, and failure of leadership, not the people performing the process. Teamwork is the key to a successful business, and the CQI process aims to encourage teamwork. As a result of satisfied staff and clients, profits tend to be positively affected. The CQI uses strategies such as brainstorming to allow for the free flow of beneficial ideas. It is also important to observe competitors in the industry to see how others address similar issues. Team

Copyright © Mometrix Media. You have been licensed one copy of this document for personal use only. Any other reproduction or redistribution is strictly prohibited. All rights reserved.
This content is provided for test preparation purposes only and does not imply an endorsement by Mometrix of any particular political, scientific, or religious point of view.

members on a CQI panel may be from all levels of staff and management working together to solve a common problem.

OT's Role

Occupational therapy departments have processes that may be passed down from year to year. From time to time a committee of occupational therapists (OTs) need to come together to discuss and review policies, protocols, and procedures. Many times, the current set of policies, protocols, and procedures are out dated and need updating. It is through the brainstorming process, discussion, and negotiation that committee members are able to agree upon new policies and procedures based upon best practices. OTs also participate in hospital-wide continuous quality improvement (CQI) committees. Certifications include those such as Lean Six Sigma. Lean Six Sigma is a method that relies on a collaborative approach to systematically remove waste and recommend a framework for overall organizational culture. Although hospitals have their own systems of quality improvement, most rely on a systematic approach such as the Lean Six Sigma system.

Service Delivery of OT Services

As regulations and service delivery demands change in the health care industry, the occupational therapy (OT) profession must be flexible to change its rules and regulations to match new demands. The continuous quality improvement (CQI) process forms a structured method to encourage the flexibility and critical thinking necessary to complete this process. OT committees frequently meet to adopt or change billing practices, paperwork, and rules regarding patient treatment in an effort to comply with federal regulations. Without the CQI process, committees would not have the organization to complete work in a fast-paced industry.

Software for Occupational Therapy Documentation

There are only a few well-known software packages available to perform occupational therapy documentation. Although some companies use software out of the box, without modifications, others have the software company make requested changes to the software. Although the fill-in-the-blank option takes much time, it is the most descriptive and accurate way of giving information. In a fast-paced environment, a lot of writing can be almost impossible. Drop-down menu items pose a more realistic method as they are still accurate but do not take as much time. Once the continuous quality improvement identifies the issue of canned software, a committee can begin working on meeting with software companies to find the best software for the clinic needs. Once the software is identified, a sample of therapists can trial and give feedback as to whether or not the software is appropriate for the clinic.

Occupational Therapy Assistant's Role in Patient Evaluation and Discharge Process

The occupational therapy assistant contributes to the screening, evaluation, and reevaluation by implementing delegated assessments and by providing verbal and written reports of observation to the occupational therapist (OT). The intervention plan is formed in collaboration with the OT. The assistant can select the intervention plan. However, the intervention should be congruent with the OT's goals. If changes to the treatment plan are warranted, the OT and assistant discuss progress and, together, plan on the next step. During the discharge, the OT and assistant collaborate to determine if goals have been met. Some occupational therapy assistants are well versed in goniometry and are able to take accurate measurements for the OT during the evaluation. Occupational therapy assistants also can observe activities of daily living skills to rate (using a measurement such as the Functional Independence Measure) for scoring.

Copyright © Mometrix Media. You have been licensed one copy of this document for personal use only. Any other reproduction or redistribution is strictly prohibited. All rights reserved.
This content is provided for test preparation purposes only and does not imply an endorsement by Mometrix of any particular political, scientific, or religious point of view.

OT's Role in Preventative Medicine

Occupational therapy plays a major role in preventative medicine as occupational therapists (OTs) understand the value in promoting health and well-being for every stage in life. The primary goal of an OT is to keep the client engaged in activities of everyday life. OTs understand how illness, injury, and disability challenge a client's way of life. OTs work in a variety of settings and do not only focus on therapy for the infirmed but also on the prevention of illness. One of the settings that OTs support is independent and assisted living centers. In these settings, OTs conduct exercise classes, water aerobics, and information sessions on a wide variety of subjects such as home safety and fall prevention. OTs are also diligent about providing home programs so that once a person has recovered from an illness, he or she is able to use an exercise program as a way to maintain strength, endurance, and overall health.

OT's Role in Advancing Positive Outcomes for Children with Autism

Occupational therapists (OTs) assist in the growth and development of children with autism. Occupational therapists are experts in social, emotional, and physiological effects of autism on the family unit. Through therapy, OTs work to train children with autism to be able to perform self-care as well as improve social interaction, behavioral, and classroom performance. OTs also train family members in the care and management of children with autism. Through increasing the basic skills of these children, many are able to function in society and lead productive lives. However, some children with autism continue to need therapy as adults. Skills such as homemaking, finances, meal preparation, taking public transportation, and laundry are typical skills OTs work on with autistic adults.

OT's Role in Advancing Positive Outcomes with the Elderly Population

Occupational therapists (OTs) perform wellness programs such as exercise and yoga at wellness centers, independent living, assisted living, and skilled living centers. Studies show that active adults are better able to stay healthy. Occupational therapy also works on cognitive skills in the same living communities in the form of games, current event groups, and outings. The OT's home assessment focuses on safety and looks for fall risks such as throw rugs, cords, uneven surfaces, and other hazards in the home. Medical alerts are also a welcome addition for many clients as they are a safety item that can be utilized in the event of a medical emergency. The home program is, perhaps, the most important aspect of a wellness program. Through the home exercise program, clients can exercise on a daily basis even when they are not actively involved in therapy.

OT's Role in Advancing Positive Outcomes with Alzheimer's Patients

Positive health outcomes are not only measured in physical health but in psychological health. As Alzheimer's disease takes its toll on both patient and caregiver, occupational therapists (OTs) are able to assist in improving daily functional skills by providing for equipment needs, training, and guidance in key areas such as bathroom safety, basic self-care needs, physical exercise, fall reduction, environmental adaptation, and caregiver support. By optimizing the client's strengths, an OT is able to assist each patient to lead life to the fullest. Positive outcomes can also come in the form of reduced emergency room visits and reduced inpatient hospital stays. As the number of hospital readmissions decreases, there is a direct correlation to the well-being of the patient and his or her ability to lead life in a healthy manner.

OT's Role in Wellness and Prevention

The Affordable Care Act (ACA) places an increased emphasis on preventing disease and injury. Occupational therapists take a holistic approach that is optimal for the prevention of disease as well as wellness programs. Occupational therapists participate in the following educational programs:

Copyright © Mometrix Media. You have been licensed one copy of this document for personal use only. Any other reproduction or redistribution is strictly prohibited. All rights reserved.
This content is provided for test preparation purposes only and does not imply an endorsement by Mometrix of any particular political, scientific, or religious point of view.

ergonomics for computers, tablets, obesity prevention, handwriting education, fall prevention, programs for car modification, child growth and development programs, universal design, environmental assessments, aging-in-place programs for seniors, training in balance, training in body mechanics, and research to promote wellness (to name a few). Occupational therapists are hired by hospitals, outpatient therapy clinics, industries, and companies to promote wellness and treat those employees as appropriate. Therapists also are hired by some companies to prevent injury as well as treat injured workers.

Safety, Emergency Response, and Risk Management

Infection Control

Infection control refers to policies and procedures used to reduce the risk of spreading infections in any health care setting. These diseases are usually caused by bacteria and viruses that can spread by human contact through touch or droplets. Hospital-acquired infections or nosocomial infections can lead to increased hospital stays, antibiotic use (and possible resistance), and even death. The use of universal precautions is aimed at avoiding getting in contact with germs and disease. Proper techniques during medical procedures as well as the proper sanitization of surgical devices are also important to maintaining good infection control. There are currently several nationally sponsored hospital programs aimed at reducing the rate of these infections as they cost the medical industry billions of dollars each year.

Universal Precautions

Universal precautions are practices to avoid exposure to bodily fluids to avoid the spread of infection. Equipment such as medical gloves, goggles, face shields, and gowns prevent bodily fluids from making contact with clothing and tissues. Under universal precautions, all patients are considered possible carriers of blood-borne pathogens. These materials, when discarded, are placed in specially marked red bags that identify the materials inside as hazardous. The red bag is usually professionally destroyed by companies that specialize in handling medical waste. In many cases, medical waste is burned. In a hospital, universal precautions are meant to be followed not only by medical staff but also by visiting family members.

Use of Universal Precautions When Working with Clients on Bathing and Dressing

Occupational therapists work with clients in self-care training. Part of that training involves assisting clients with bathing and dressing. One has to always assume that there may be blood-borne pathogens on articles of clothing, bathroom equipment, and grooming supplies. The best universal precaution to use is to wear gloves. This forms a barrier between you and the client (and clothing). Therapists will often wear a gown when assisting a client to bathe as this prevents the splashing of bodily fluids and water to get on the therapist's clothing. No matter how or what you do to maintain universal precautions, it is important to use an alcohol gel or soap to clean hands after any type of patient treatment. Good hand hygiene and proper infection control techniques are both important methods to stop the spread of infections.

Precautions for Blood-Borne Pathogens

Blood-borne pathogens most commonly found in the health care industry are diseases like human immunodeficiency virus, hepatitis B, and hepatitis C. These pathogens are transmitted through blood, semen, and vaginal secretions. Exposure occurs if the skin is broken such as from a needle stick or other sharp object. When occupational therapists perform activities or activities of daily living with these patients, it is very important to wear a gown, gloves, and face shield if there is any

Copyright © Mometrix Media. You have been licensed one copy of this document for personal use only. Any other reproduction or redistribution is strictly prohibited. All rights reserved.
This content is provided for test preparation purposes only and does not imply an endorsement by Mometrix of any particular political, scientific, or religious point of view.

risk of bodily fluids splashing and reaching the therapist. Good hand washing skills are imperative after working with clients with these diseases. If exposure occurs, report it at once to your supervisor. Treatment may be recommended and will need to be initiated as soon as possible.

Precautions for Patients with *C. Diff*

Clostridioides difficile (*C. Diff*) spores are transmitted by touch and affect the gastrointestinal tract, causing inflammation of the colon and diarrhea. A person with this bacterium is on long-term antibiotics. This is very contagious and requires the patient to be in contact isolation. This means the patient should be treated in his or her room. People entering the patient's room are given a gown, shoe covers, and gloves so that the spores from this disease do not get on the clothing and shoes. All items that make contact with this patient need to be sanitized after use. The gown, shoe covers, and gloves are removed after leaving the room and thrown away in a special waste container set outside the patient's room. Staff need to thoroughly wash their hands after leaving the patient's room.

Disinfecting Equipment Between Patients

Cross contamination of germs is a very big concern in the medical community. Many rehab facilities have equipment that is used throughout the whole day. This means sound infection control principles need to be enforced. Items handled by patients need to be sprayed and left to air dry or wiped down with a hospital-grade germicide. Most germicides must be allowed to air dry as this gives the chemicals a chance to kill germs. There are some items, such as paraffin, that cannot be disinfected and should be discarded after each use. Once a day, it is also important to wipe down doorknobs, handles, tabletops, and chairs as these items are places patients and therapists touch and can also contain germs. Infection control standards change, depending upon hospital policy and government policies; it is important to remain informed and flexible to maintain good infection control techniques.

Standard Diagnostic Equipment Stored in Patient Rehab Gym for Medical Emergencies

Most rehab gyms have access to at least one stethoscope, blood pressure cuff, pulse oximeter, various size gloves, face shield, gown, hand sanitizer, sanitizing soap, spill kit, bleach, and a standard first aid kit containing Band-Aids, antibiotic ointment, gauze, tweezers, ace wrap, and a cold pack. If the rehab gym is free standing, it may be necessary to carry more equipment. However, if the gym is part of a hospital, some equipment may be accessible at a nearby first aid station. Larger gyms or gyms with multiple rooms may need more than one of each item. Look to administrative departments to provide guidance based on corporate policies.

Reaction When Patient Gets Dizzy During a Standing Activity

Depending upon the patient's diagnosis and medical history, there could be several causes for dizziness. The first thing to do is to sit the patient down. The second thing to do is to take the patient's blood pressure and pulse. Observe skin color, whether the patient becomes diaphoretic, or if the dizziness does not pass. If you are in a health care setting, call a nurse. If you are in the patient's home, stop activities until the symptoms subside. If the symptoms persist, it may be necessary (especially if blood pressure is elevated) to call the physician's office or 911. If the symptoms subside and the patient wants to resume therapy, do an activity or light exercise while sitting. Continue monitoring vital signs periodically.

Copyright © Mometrix Media. You have been licensed one copy of this document for personal use only. Any other reproduction or redistribution is strictly prohibited. All rights reserved.
This content is provided for test preparation purposes only and does not imply an endorsement by Mometrix of any particular political, scientific, or religious point of view.

Course of Action if Patient Has Severe Pain in Back of Knee and Swelling Below the Knee

The most common cause of posterior knee pain in combination with leg swelling is a blood clot. Therefore, suspend all therapy, and notify the nurse and/or doctor. Do not attempt to walk the patient to his or her room as increased activity and heart rate put the patient at risk for the blood clot dislodging and traveling to the lungs or brain. Also, do not place hot packs over this area as heat can increase circulation and also dislodge a blood clot. It may be necessary for the doctor to order a doppler ultrasound to rule out a blood clot. If all is clear, activity most likely will be resumed by the doctor. If there is a blood clot, clot-dissolving drugs will be given to the patient.

Course of Action if Total Hip Replacement Patient Complains of Increasing Pain in the Operated Hip

An orthopedic patient who complains of hip pain after hip replacement surgery is very common. However, new pain could mean hardware is out of place or the hip joint is not fitting correctly. The best course of action is to discontinue therapy until the nurse and doctor examine the patient. In most cases, the doctor will order an X-ray to determine alignment of the joint. If the joint is unstable, surgical repair may be necessary. However, if the joint looks good, most likely therapy will be resumed. It is always good to have a discussion with a patient to determine pain level prior to therapy. On days when the pain level is higher, a lighter therapy session is beneficial. This type of discussion helps avoid over exercising the patient.

Course of Action if Post Stroke Patient Becomes Unusually Confused During Treatment Session

If a patient has a new onset of dizziness, the first thing to do is to have the patient sit or lay down. Next, take the patient's blood pressure. If the blood pressure is normal, continue monitoring the patient and call the nurse or doctor's office (if in an outpatient setting). If the blood pressure is high, monitor the patient and have someone call the nurse or 911 (if an in an outpatient clinic). These symptoms may be related to the previous stroke, or they may be signs of a new stroke. Therefore, time is of the essence. There are occasions during which you may be the only one in the clinic and do not have the availability of a second person to assist with an emergency. In this event, it is important to call the nurse or 911 as soon as the patient is sitting or lying down.

Safety Measures for Cooking Activity Involving High-Level Patients with Varying Diagnoses

There are a few safety measures that should be implemented when performing kitchen activities with a patient or a group of patients. Always have a fire extinguisher present when performing a kitchen task. Make sure tripping hazards are removed from the pathways necessary to retrieve items from places like the refrigerator, cabinets, pantry, oven, and stovetop. It is also important to make sure that the cooking activity fits the allotted time for the treatment. Rushing to complete a complex activity, due to lack of time, can cause injuries such as cuts, burns, and falls. If more than one patient is involved in the activity, it may be necessary to have an additional therapist or aide present for safety.

Performing Mat Activities in Sitting Position with Stroke Patient with Balance Deficits

Balance activities in a sitting position are essential to perform at the mat level to facilitate movement, righting reactions, weight bearing to modulate tone, as well as activity tolerance. However, there should always be two people assisting in the treatment of this type of patient. One person usually assists the patient to maintain balance, while the second person assists the patient

Copyright © Mometrix Media. You have been licensed one copy of this document for personal use only. Any other reproduction or redistribution is strictly prohibited. All rights reserved.
This content is provided for test preparation purposes only and does not imply an endorsement by Mometrix of any particular political, scientific, or religious point of view.

to perform the activity. The patient is usually guarded from the back or side to prevent falling. Make sure the patient's hips are situated away from the edge of the mat and feet are flat on the floor to prevent forward loss of balance. When reaching activities are performed from side to side, the patient may need to be guarded by two people on either side of the patient, while the third person performs the activity from in front of the patient.

TRANSFERRING A PATIENT IN A TOTAL ASSIST FROM BED TO WHEELCHAIR

A patient who needs a total assist with transfers requires two people. This is a safety precaution to be used no matter what method of transfers is used. The safest method of transferring this patient will be to use a mechanical lift. However, if you are incorporating any balance, bedside activities, or activities of daily living into the treatment, then a two-person lift may be possible (although not the preferred method). Prepare all materials used for the transfer prior to starting to work with the patient as it is difficult to interrupt a transfer. A cooperative patient always makes the transfer easier. Explain to the patient what will be happening during the transfer so that they are prepared and know what to expect. Transfers can be traumatic for patients. Therefore, talk to the patient during the transfer in a reassuring voice so that he or she is better able to keep calm and reassured.

TREATING A PTSD PATIENT WHO IS NERVOUS AROUND PEOPLE

Patients with posttraumatic stress disorder (PTSD) are sometimes nervous around other people. It will be best to treat this patient in a quiet, non-busy environment. For some people this may mean a secluded room. Other patients may prefer staying in their room for therapy. There may even be some patients who are willing to come to the rehab gym as long as treatment is scheduled at times the gym has fewer patients. It is best to discuss these options prior to the first treatment. This patient may also be reluctant to engage in activities. Be sure to agree on goals and treatment approaches with this patient. It will be important to gain this patient's trust early on in the therapy process. If a negative treatment experience does occur, give the patient space and time to recover. Allow him to come back to therapy when ready.

Laws, Regulations, Accreditation, and Reimbursement

FINDING FACILITY POLICIES RELATED TO OCCUPATIONAL THERAPY

Facility policies relating to the practice of occupational therapy can be found in a few places. First, online versions of most policies can be found on most facility websites. This can be accessed by most intranet sites from a facility computer. A hard copy of most, if not all, policies is stored in most therapy departments. Finally, employees are usually required to take online education courses through the facility's intranet. These courses usually have a section on basic company policies. As policies are updated, it is up to management to inform employees of those updates. Many managers will email new or updated policies to employees. Policies related to safety (such as Material Safety Data Sheets) should be stored in an accessible place that can be easily retrieved in the event of an emergency.

FINDING NATIONAL AND STATE GUIDELINES FOR PRACTICE OF OTS

There are several sources on the Internet that state the federal and national guidelines. The American Occupational Therapy Association has guidelines regarding all federal requirements. Guidelines are divided into the categories of continuing competence, licensure requirements, the regulation of OTs, supervision of OTs/OT assistants/aides/students, and telehealth. Each state has its own guidelines that OTs need to become familiar with prior to applying for an initial license and when reapplying for licensure renewal. Federal guidelines tend to be more general, whereas state guidelines are specific to the practice of OTs within that state. For the OT to obtain a renewal

Copyright © Mometrix Media. You have been licensed one copy of this document for personal use only. Any other reproduction or redistribution is strictly prohibited. All rights reserved.
This content is provided for test preparation purposes only and does not imply an endorsement by Mometrix of any particular political, scientific, or religious point of view.

license, a jurisprudence test, covering state guidelines, needs to be passed with a minimum score that varies depending upon the state

Finding Accreditation Guidelines for Outpatient Facilities

The American Occupational Therapy Association (AOTA) has a brief summary of accreditation guidelines for outpatient facilities listed on its website. However, the best place to research accreditation guidelines is from the source, The Centers for Medicare and Medicaid Services (CMS). CMS has the guidelines divided into those for each state, outpatient rehabilitation providers, and enforcement guidelines of quality, safety, and oversight. Some occupational therapists are in charge of outpatient clinics and will need to have a working knowledge of these guidelines. Facilities have to renew their licenses periodically with the state and are challenged with the task of keeping up with the time frames for renewals as well as compliance with regulations.

Finding Required Supervision for a COTA

The levels of supervision for a certified occupational therapy assistant (COTA) vary from state to state. Occupational therapists and COTAs are required to know the types and frequency of supervision for the state in which they are licensed to practice. Each state has slightly different guidelines. As guidelines change, licensing boards typically send out a copy of these changes to facilities as well as licensees. Therapy facilities are obligated to follow state guidelines. However, some facilities also have additional regulations regarding the practice of COTAs. Each therapist should be introduced, by his or her supervisor, to facility guidelines for practice and where to find an electronic or written copy of those guidelines.

Concepts of Skilled Service and Medically Necessary

Occupational therapy is a skilled service. That means the treatment received in occupational therapy cannot be delivered by family members, other therapy team members, nurses, or physicians. Medically necessary means that the patient requires training in the skilled services that occupational therapists are trained to deliver. Once the goals of the patient are achieved or the patient, for other reasons, does not require skilled occupational therapy services, he or she is discharged from occupational therapy. At this point, a home program is usually administered so accomplishments from therapy can be continued post therapy treatment. Medically necessary means that the patient has had a significant change in health status, usually from disease or injury, to warrant occupational therapy services. Additionally, chronic illness can also cause a decline in health status and warrant occupational therapy services.

Reimbursement Policies

Reimbursement policies refers to those conditions that have to be met for insurance companies to pay for therapy services. Most insurance companies follow Medicare guidelines and require that occupational therapy (OT) documentation for services provided show evidence of being skilled and medically necessary. The documentation guidelines are very detailed. Generally, the evaluation needs to be thorough with measurable short- and long-term goals. Therapists need to document progress in treatment notes as well as progress notes to be considered for reimbursement. Reimbursement usually stops once the patient has reached a point in which therapy services are not warranted (meaning not requiring skilled or medically necessary services). OT departments are very conscious of newer and stricter OT reimbursement guidelines over the past several years as denials for reimbursement have increased.

Copyright © Mometrix Media. You have been licensed one copy of this document for personal use only. Any other reproduction or redistribution is strictly prohibited. All rights reserved.
This content is provided for test preparation purposes only and does not imply an endorsement by Mometrix of any particular political, scientific, or religious point of view.

Influence of Medicare Reimbursement Policies and Skilled and Necessary Services on Occupational Therapy Services

Skilled Nursing Facility

In a skilled nursing facility, Medicare will reimburse for occupational therapy services at 100% for the first 20 days. From day 21 to 100, Medicare will pay 80% and the patient will pay 20%. If the patient has a co-insurance, the co-insurance will usually pay the remaining 20%. After day 100, Medicare will not reimburse for skilled therapy. If a person completes therapy in a skilled facility and has to later return due to a new illness, the reimbursement cycle starts from the beginning. Therefore, each 100-day episode is related to a specific illness. With the Medicare reimbursement days limited, it is very important for occupational therapists to be cognizant of treating a patient for only that period of time that services are deemed skilled and medically necessary.

Home Health

Medicare requires a person receiving home health to be homebound. This means it would require a significant and taxing effort for the patient to leave home. Medicare authorizes therapy services (occupational, physical, and speech therapy) for intervals of 60 days at a time. The way therapy services work in home health is very complicated. Basically, home health companies receive a basic reimbursement based upon patient diagnosis and medical/functional level; this money is then divided among each discipline providing services. Therefore, no single discipline can see a patient for the full 60 days. All disciplines that see the patient have to, generally, limit their time to 2 to 3 weeks with the patient. Occasionally, occupational therapy may be the only home health therapy discipline. In this case, the patient may be seen for up to 4 to 6 weeks.

Importance of Monitoring Outcomes for Therapy Services

As patients are discharged from occupational therapy services, the occupational therapist determines whether or not the patient met the long-term goals. Over a period of time, the outcomes of the long-term goals met as well as unmet are tracked among therapists. Therapist also can determine if goals are consistently under- or overstated. The monitoring of outcomes occurs during the chart audit process. Medicare tracks similar outcomes among facilities. The purpose of tracking outcomes is to learn which areas of service need improvement. Medicare publishes outcomes so that the public can view which facilities are better rated for patient care. Outcomes are usually measured on a monthly, quarterly, and yearly basis.

Uniformed Terminology

Uniformed Terminology is a document that is published by the American Occupational Therapy Association that explains the areas of practice for occupational therapy (OT). The document is divided in to two sections—performance areas and performance components. Performance areas include activities of daily living, work, play, or leisure. These areas are typically part of daily life. Performance components are the elements of performance necessary to be successful in the performance areas. These components consist of sensorimotor, cognitive, psychosocial, and psychological areas. Uniformed Terminology is a way of unifying the purpose and role of OT into terms that are understandable to the public and are consistent with the goals of OT. It is also the method for which the profession of OT defines itself.

Using Standard Approved Abbreviations for Documentation

There are hundreds of abbreviations that have become standard as part of documentation in occupational therapy. However, it is up to each facility to determine which abbreviations will be adopted for use in documentation. Some abbreviations are not used because they can have multiple meanings depending upon which discipline is writing the documentation. Some abbreviations are

Copyright © Mometrix Media. You have been licensed one copy of this document for personal use only. Any other reproduction or redistribution is strictly prohibited. All rights reserved.
This content is provided for test preparation purposes only and does not imply an endorsement by Mometrix of any particular political, scientific, or religious point of view.

confusing and also have not been accepted by facilities. It is important for the occupational therapist to learn and keep a list of standard abbreviations approved by his or her facility. Also, many computerized medical records will not recognize unapproved abbreviations. Medical abbreviations are not used when communicating to patients and family members. Medical terms are described in simple-to-understand terms.

Importance of Peer-Reviewed Chart Audit Process

The chart audit process is important to a department to determine timeliness, quality, and outcomes of documentation. Although many supervisors perform chart audits, it is also customary for therapists to audit each other's work. The chart audit form is usually completed online so that it can be tracked using a spreadsheet. This is also how infection control, timeliness of documentation, thoroughness of documentation, and outcomes of goals are tracked. The chart audit is usually reported to the quality management team at most facilities. The quality management team will then review chart audit results and make quality improvement recommendations for the rehab department. Facilities are also required to report certain outcomes to Medicare. In turn, Medicare uses these numbers to track national trends.

Professional Development and Standards

Service Competency

Service competency is a set of basic skills required to perform a job efficiently. In health care service competency usually involves the following attributes: patient-centered care, interdisciplinary teamwork, evidence-based practice, quality improvement, and utilizing information technology. All of the basic attributes of service competency are interdependent. In other words, it is difficult to perform patient-centered care without conferring with other members of the team (interdisciplinary teamwork). Likewise, much of the decision-making process regarding a patient's care hinges upon evidence-based practice. Evidence-based practice is the result of scholarly research and articles that are shared through the Internet (information technology). Health care relies upon the intricacies of information technology to record and share patient information with medical professionals, insurance companies, and federal agencies. At the center of these five competencies is the patient. All competencies must be with the patient in mind.

Professional Development

Health care professionals are continually learning new information regarding their practice specialties. Continuing education is required in every discipline. However, the number of hours required are only set at a minimum for license renewal. Professional development can take many forms such as live seminars, webinars, printed courses, and advanced degrees. Within a hospital, there are also opportunities for professional development within the workplace. Additionally, many hospitals offer grand rounds, in-services, and seminars for employees. Professional development is a lifelong commitment that does not stop with a degree or a management position. As research and new discoveries are made in medicine, it is up to each professional to keep up with those discoveries that would benefit their therapy practice. Each professional is also left with the decision as to which courses or seminars are best for his or her current mix of patients.

Identifying Need for Professional Development

The job appraisal process is one method to identify current competencies as well as the need for further education. During the job appraisal process, each employee performs a self-assessment. This self-assessment is very similar to the appraisal the employee receives from a supervisor. The supervisor is then able to see the responses from the employee and integrate his or her goals with

Copyright © Mometrix Media. You have been licensed one copy of this document for personal use only. Any other reproduction or redistribution is strictly prohibited. All rights reserved.
This content is provided for test preparation purposes only and does not imply an endorsement by Mometrix of any particular political, scientific, or religious point of view.

departmental expectations. The result is a set of professional development goals that have been created by a collaboration of the employee and supervisor. These goals also help establish a career path for the employee. Although goals can be changed, this is a starting point to gain knowledge in weaker areas or to bolster current knowledge. The end goal is quality patient care.

Occupational Therapy Standards of Practice

This document defines minimum standards for practicing occupational therapists (OTs). These standards of practice are essential for OTs and OT assistants in the delivery of services as they define the expectations and roles for both OTs and OT assistants. The document is divided into several sections. The first section describes educational requirements. The next section, professional standing and responsibility, sets the standard for maintaining licensure and providing a safe client environment. The next section lays out the standards for screenings, evaluations, and reevaluations. The third section describes ethical considerations in providing and documenting interventions. The final section describes the OT's and assistant's roles in documenting outcomes to intervention and family training. These documents provide a framework from which states define more specific roles of the OT and OT assistant.

Occupational Therapy Code of Conduct

The standards of conduct define and clarify the standards of personal and professional conduct required for eligibility for both initial and continued certification. The governing body for this is the National Board for Certification in Occupational Therapy. There are nine principles that make up the code of conduct. These subsections have to do with the timely and truthful submission of information requested, cooperation during compliance review, the integrity of answering communications to the board, compliance of state laws, reporting convictions, not engaging in harmful behavior, not misusing the national board's intellectual properties, and not engaging in occupational therapy practice if judgement is impaired.

Copyright © Mometrix Media. You have been licensed one copy of this document for personal use only. Any other reproduction or redistribution is strictly prohibited. All rights reserved.
This content is provided for test preparation purposes only and does not imply an endorsement by Mometrix of any particular political, scientific, or religious point of view.

NBCOT Practice Test

Want to take this practice test in an online interactive format?
Check out the online resources page, which includes interactive practice questions and much more: **mometrix.com/resources719/ota**

1. The National Board of Certification in Occupational Therapy (NBCOT) has established a Code of Professional Conduct that guides the practice of occupational therapy. Which statement is consistent with the Code of Professional Conduct?

a. A COTA must disclose any criminal, legal, or disciplinary matters to NBCOT within 90 days of occurrence.
b. A COTA must disclose any criminal, legal, or disciplinary matters to NBCOT within 30 days of occurrence.
c. A COTA must disclose any criminal, legal, or disciplinary matters to NBCOT within 60 days of occurrence.

2. A patient has been referred to occupational therapy (OT) with a diagnosis of secondary rotator cuff impingement. The OT plan of care indicates that the patient should be instructed in a home exercise program to address the associated muscle weakness. Which muscles would be MOST appropriate to address in the initial home exercise program?

Select the three (3) best choices.

a. Supraspinatus
b. Lower trapezius
c. Infraspinatus
d. Rhomboid major
e. Serratus anterior
f. Teres minor

3. Which areas are the MOST high risk for pressure injuries for a wheelchair-bound patient who is seated in a standard manual wheelchair with footrests and cannot perform pressure-relieving techniques?

Select the three (3) best choices.

a. Lateral malleolus
b. Olecranon process
c. Ischial tuberosity
d. Vertebral spinous process
e. Head of fibula
f. Lateral condyle of femur

Copyright © Mometrix Media. You have been licensed one copy of this document for personal use only. Any other reproduction or redistribution is strictly prohibited. All rights reserved.
This content is provided for test preparation purposes only and does not imply an endorsement by Mometrix of any particular political, scientific, or religious point of view.

4. A COTA is treating a patient who is on isolation precautions due to an MRSA infection in a right forearm wound. The COTA is scheduled to perform bilateral upper extremity range of motion exercises with the patient at bedside. Which protective equipment is required to be worn by the COTA?

a. Gloves and gown
b. Mask and gloves
c. Respirator, gown, and gloves
d. Mask, gloves, and gown

5. Which instructions would be MOST appropriate for a patient in the active inflammatory period of rheumatoid arthritis?

a. Limit stretching exercises to gentle stretches of brief duration.
b. Perform isometric exercises in pain-free positions.
c. Limit exercise performance to one session per day.
d. Perform low-intensity resistance exercises through pain-free range of motion.

6. Which technique would be the LEAST effective means for communicating instructions to a child with autism?

a. Provide both verbal and visual information to the child.
b. Get the child's attention, then provide verbal information.
c. Provide instruction in the form of a two-step command.

7. A long-term care resident fell while transferring from a wheelchair to the toilet with the nursing staff and sprained his right ankle. His doctor has written occupational therapy orders for the patient. Which factor best supports the medical necessity for occupational therapy intervention?

a. The patient requires moderate assistance to transfer from a wheelchair to the toilet.
b. Since the fall, the patient's right ankle has been swollen and painful.
c. The patient requires minimal assistance with clothes management during toileting.
d. Since the fall, the patient requires a higher level of assistance for toilet transfers than previously.

8. A client is noted to be routine oriented, prefers to be alone, and dislikes crowds. Which sensory pattern best describes this client?

a. Bystander
b. Seeker
c. Avoider
d. Sensor

9. The occupational therapy plan of care indicates that a wrist support brace should be fabricated to maintain the hand in the functional position. Which positions are correct for the splint fabrication?

Select the three (3) best choices.

a. Twenty degrees of wrist extension
b. Twenty degrees of wrist flexion
c. Slight radial deviation
d. Slight ulnar deviation
e. Thirty degrees of metacarpal flexion
f. Sixty degrees of metacarpal flexion

Copyright © Mometrix Media. You have been licensed one copy of this document for personal use only. Any other reproduction or redistribution is strictly prohibited. All rights reserved.
This content is provided for test preparation purposes only and does not imply an endorsement by Mometrix of any particular political, scientific, or religious point of view.

10. An employer has requested that an occupational therapy job analysis be performed as part of the pre-employment screening process for all new hires. Which type of job analysis would be MOST appropriate?

a. Functional
b. Occupation based
c. Risk assessment

11. A 60-year-old client who is 4 months status-post bilateral total knee replacements has been referred to occupational therapy for instruction in proper lifting technique, so he can return to his job as a stocker at a grocery store. Which lift technique would be MOST appropriate for this client?

a. One-leg stance
b. Deep squat
c. Stoop
d. Half kneeling

12. A 60-year-old female with an acute exacerbation of chronic obstructive pulmonary disease (COPD) is being discharged home from the acute care hospital. Her home setup includes a combination tub shower. Her goal is to be able to shower with supervision from her husband. Which assistive device will she MOST likely require for bathing?

a. Long-handled sponge
b. Tub seat
c. Grab bar

13. Which statements best describe evidence-based practice in occupational therapy?

Select the three (3) best choices.

a. Treatment is guided by up-to-date research and scientific information.
b. The client is actively involved in the intervention process.
c. Personal clinical experience does not factor into evidence-based practice.
d. Research and scientific information should be directly related to occupational therapy principles.
e. Evidence-based practice highly values the use of diagnosis-based protocols for treatment.
f. The first step in implementing evidence-based practice is to formulate a clinical question.

14. Which type of research study provides the BEST source for evidence-based practice?

a. Descriptive studies
b. Randomized controlled trials
c. Nonexperimental studies
d. Systematic review

15. Which muscles are MOST likely to develop contractures after a transfemoral amputation?

a. Hip flexors and hamstrings
b. Hip flexors and hip abductors
c. Hip flexors and hip adductors

Copyright © Mometrix Media. You have been licensed one copy of this document for personal use only. Any other reproduction or redistribution is strictly prohibited. All rights reserved.
This content is provided for test preparation purposes only and does not imply an endorsement by Mometrix of any particular political, scientific, or religious point of view.

16. The occupational therapy evaluation states that a child tested positive for gravitational insecurity. Which clinical observation MOST accurately describes gravitational insecurity?

a. The child has difficulty stabilizing the shoulders, neck, arms, and trunk as the occupational therapist attempts to move the child.
b. The child has difficulty sitting on a large therapy ball while the occupational therapist tips the ball from side to side.
c. The child has difficulty lifting the head, neck, and trunk against gravity while in the prone position.
d. The child has difficulty lying supine on a large therapy ball while the occupational therapist tips the ball backward unexpectedly.

17. During normal development, which oral motor reflex diminishes at 2 years of age?

a. Rooting
b. Sucking
c. Biting
d. Gagging

18. Which feeding skill typically develops around 12 months of age?

a. The jaw remains stable for tongue and lip movements and for control with chewing.
b. The ability to move food from side to side in the mouth develops.
c. The upper lip moves down when being spoon-fed.

19. An interdisciplinary oral motor/feeding group is being planned for children with refusal-to-eat feeding issues. The COTA is planning activities for the children for the first week of the feeding group. Which treatment approach is the LEAST likely to be successful for the children in this group during the first week?

a. Doing art projects with food
b. Encouraging the children to share their food
c. Allowing the children to help prepare the snack
d. Playing pretend food games

20. Which self-feeding strategy would be MOST effective for a patient with macular degeneration?

a. Putting food on the plate using the clock method
b. Turning the head to compensate for visual deficits
c. Dimming the lights in the room

21. Which condition would be a contraindication for cryotherapy?

a. Raynaud's phenomenon
b. Chronic obstructive pulmonary disease
c. Acute ankle sprain
d. Systemic lupus erythematosus

22. Which condition is the MOST likely to be treated with serial casting to address restricted range of motion?

a. Heterotopic ossification
b. Scarring from burns
c. Neurological spasticity

Copyright © Mometrix Media. You have been licensed one copy of this document for personal use only. Any other reproduction or redistribution is strictly prohibited. All rights reserved.
This content is provided for test preparation purposes only and does not imply an endorsement by Mometrix of any particular political, scientific, or religious point of view.

23. The occupational therapy (OT) plan of care for a patient with cardiac precautions indicates that OT activities should not exceed the light metabolic equivalent (MET) level. Which therapeutic activities would this patient be allowed to perform?

Select the three (3) best choices.

a. Upper extremity bicycling
b. Washing dishes
c. Knitting
d. Putting away groceries
e. Preparing a family dinner
f. Walking on a treadmill at 2.5 mph

24. A COTA is performing a therapeutic exercise with a patient with a complete T6 spinal cord injury in an inpatient rehabilitation setting. The patient suddenly complains of a severe headache. He is also noted to have goosebumps on his arms, and his face is flushed. What are the correct actions for the COTA to take in this situation?

Select the three (3) best choices.

a. Monitor the patient for 15 minutes to see if the symptoms resolve.
b. Call for immediate medical assistance.
c. Lie the patient down flat in the supine position.
d. Decrease the intensity of the exercise.
e. Look for any noxious stimulation that may be the cause of his distress.
f. Attempt to position the patient in a seated position.

25. A patient sustained a deep partial-thickness burn that runs from his right distal upper arm to his distal lower arm. Which elbow and forearm motions will MOST likely be restricted?

a. Elbow extension and forearm supination
b. Elbow flexion and forearm supination
c. Elbow extension and forearm pronation
d. Elbow flexion and forearm pronation

26. A 6-month-old baby is noted to be delayed in reaching developmental milestones. The mother is requesting information about her baby's eligibility to qualify for services to address the developmental delay. Which resource would be most relevant in this situation?

a. Individuals with Disabilities Education Act (IDEA), part A
b. Individuals with Disabilities Education Act (IDEA), part B
c. Individuals with Disabilities Education Act (IDEA), part C
d. Individuals with Disabilities Education Act (IDEA), part D

27. A 75-year-old patient has been referred for outpatient occupational therapy by his physician. Which part of his Medicare policy will cover these services?

a. Part A
b. Part B
c. Part C
d. Part D

Copyright © Mometrix Media. You have been licensed one copy of this document for personal use only. Any other reproduction or redistribution is strictly prohibited. All rights reserved.
This content is provided for test preparation purposes only and does not imply an endorsement by Mometrix of any particular political, scientific, or religious point of view.

28. Which language perception dysfunction usually results from a right hemisphere lesion of the brain?

a. Asymbolia
b. Alexia
c. Aprosodia

29. A patient picks up her hairbrush and attempts to brush her teeth. When questioned, she indicates that she wants to brush her hair. This is an example of which perceptual motor dysfunction?

a. Ideational apraxia
b. Ideomotor apraxia I
c. Ideomotor apraxia II
d. Dressing apraxia

30. A patient with a traumatic brain injury is being treated in an inpatient rehabilitation center. He is noted to be extremely agitated and confused. Which Rancho Level most appropriately describes this patient?

a. Level III
b. Level IV
c. Level V

31. The occupational therapy (OT) staff in a skilled nursing facility notice that patients are often late for the first OT session of the day, which is scheduled at 8:00 a.m. They brought the issue to the attention of the rehab director. Which action would be the most appropriate way for the rehab director to address this concern?

a. Meet with the supervisor of the nutrition department to request that breakfast trays are delivered earlier than the current schedule.
b. Meet with the nursing supervisor to discuss staffing concerns related to the number of nursing assistants who are available to assist patients with dressing and transfers between 7 a.m. and 8 a.m.
c. Report the concern to the chief compliance officer as a breach of compliance with standards of performance.
d. Bring the concern to the quality improvement committee, brainstorm possible solutions, devise a plan for change, and monitor the outcome.

32. A patient with cognitive difficulties is participating in occupational therapy (OT). The plan of care includes cognitive retraining. The OT has instructed the COTA to grade the cognitive retraining activities according to the patient's progress. Which modification would be appropriate as the patient's cognitive status improves?

a. Alter the social demands by placing the patient in a group setting.
b. Change the task to one that is more familiar to the patient.
c. Progress from internal cues to external cues.

Copyright © Mometrix Media. You have been licensed one copy of this document for personal use only. Any other reproduction or redistribution is strictly prohibited. All rights reserved.
This content is provided for test preparation purposes only and does not imply an endorsement by Mometrix of any particular political, scientific, or religious point of view.

33. A patient has been referred to occupational therapy with a diagnosis of impaired cognitive functioning due to a recent stroke. The desired outcome of the cognitive retraining session is to promote effective reasoning and problem-solving. They are working on the task of toilet transfers in a confined space. The patient performs the transfer by propelling the wheelchair through the bathroom door, locking the wheelchair brakes, and then ambulating 5 feet to the toilet. Which step of problem-solving does this scenario BEST describe?

a. Developing possible solutions
b. Choosing one best solution
c. Executing the solution
d. Evaluating the outcome

34. Which equipment is MOST appropriate for a patient with a complete C4 spinal cord injury?

Select the three (3) best choices.

a. Head control devices
b. U-cuff
c. Mouth stick
d. Postural support devices
e. Hand controls
f. Manual wheelchair

35. Which splint would be utilized by a client who is status-post flexor tendon repair surgery?

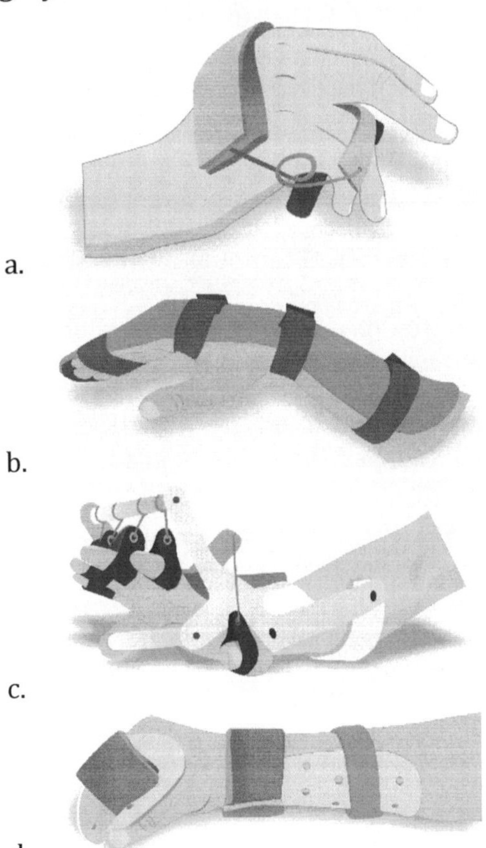

Copyright © Mometrix Media. You have been licensed one copy of this document for personal use only. Any other reproduction or redistribution is strictly prohibited. All rights reserved.
This content is provided for test preparation purposes only and does not imply an endorsement by Mometrix of any particular political, scientific, or religious point of view.

36. At the time of the initial occupational therapy evaluation, a client displayed poor– right shoulder extensor strength. At the reassessment, right shoulder extensor strength improved to fair+. What is the proper progression of exercise in this scenario with regard to client positioning?

a. Initially, exercise should be initiated in the supine position then progressed to the prone position.
b. Initially, exercise should be initiated in the prone position then progressed to the left side-lying position.
c. Initially, exercise should be initiated in the right side-lying position then progressed to the prone position.
d. Initially, exercise should be initiated in the left side-lying position then progressed to the prone position.

37. A 60-year-old construction worker with diabetes was injured 1 month ago in a work-related accident, resulting in bilateral transfemoral amputations. He has not worked since the accident and is concerned about his ability to financially support his family. Which assessment would be MOST appropriate to facilitate return to gainful employment for this client?

a. Job demands analysis
b. Functional capacity evaluation
c. Vocational evaluation

38. A person automatically places his car keys in the same location every day. Which performance pattern BEST describes this activity?

a. Roles
b. Rituals
c. Habits
d. Routines

39. Which diagnoses would MOST likely benefit from a thumb spica orthosis?

Select the three (3) best choices.

a. Median nerve injury
b. Radial nerve palsy
c. Rheumatoid arthritis
d. Cerebrovascular accident
e. De Quervain's tendinitis
f. Carpal tunnel syndrome

40. An occupational plan of care focuses on a client's occupation and associated performance skills. Which practice approach is being utilized?

a. Biomechanics
b. Motor learning
c. Rehabilitation

41. Which type of exercise is MOST likely to cause a sudden increase in blood pressure?

a. Concentric
b. Isometric
c. Eccentric

Copyright © Mometrix Media. You have been licensed one copy of this document for personal use only. Any other reproduction or redistribution is strictly prohibited. All rights reserved.
This content is provided for test preparation purposes only and does not imply an endorsement by Mometrix of any particular political, scientific, or religious point of view.

42. A patient with cognitive impairments is being taught to button a shirt. The COTA initially has the patient practice on a button board then advances the patient to buttoning his own shirt. Which remedial treatment approach is being utilized in this scenario?

a. Neurodevelopmental
b. Sensory-integration
c. Transfer-of-learning

43. A COTA in a private practice setting is filming a brief video to demonstrate a new therapeutic technique that she would like to share with her colleagues. Which statement is true with regard to the Health Insurance Portability and Accountability Act (HIPAA) and the Occupational Therapy Code of Conduct?

a. The COTA may post the video on YouTube as long as any clients in the background of the video are not named.
b. The COTA may not post the video on YouTube if clients can be seen in the background.
c. The COTA may video herself treating a client and show the video to her colleagues but may not upload the video to YouTube.

44. Which signs and symptoms are associated with an insulin reaction?

Select the three (3) best choices.

a. Labored breathing
b. Moist tongue
c. Vomiting
d. Hunger
e. Pale skin
f. Fruity breath

45. A COTA is working with a client who is exhibiting signs of shock. Which action would be MOST appropriate for the COTA to perform?

a. Place the patient in a seated position, and provide support with pillows.
b. Place the patient in the supine position, with the head slightly lower than legs.
c. Place the patient in the side-lying position, and apply a warm blanket.

46. A COTA is preparing to take a client in a wheelchair to the occupational therapy gym in a skilled nursing facility. Which action is MOST important if the client has a urinary catheter?

a. Stretch the drainage tube to make sure the tube is not kinked.
b. Empty the catheter bag if it is half-full.
c. Keep the catheter bag below the level of the bladder.

47. Which statement is true with regard to interprofessional collaboration?

a. Interprofessional collaboration creates a learning opportunity for the professionals.
b. Interprofessional collaboration utilizes a profession-centered team approach.
c. Interprofessional collaboration allows for cross-training of professional staff.

Copyright © Mometrix Media. You have been licensed one copy of this document for personal use only. Any other reproduction or redistribution is strictly prohibited. All rights reserved.
This content is provided for test preparation purposes only and does not imply an endorsement by Mometrix of any particular political, scientific, or religious point of view.

48. Which roles may be carried out by a COTA?

Select the three (3) best choices.

a. Administration of parts of a screening under an occupational therapist's supervision
b. Interpretation of the data from the occupational therapist's evaluation processes
c. Administration of select evaluation processes as determined by the supervising occupational therapist
d. Supervision of a therapy aide for delegated client-related task as determined by the occupational therapist
e. Selection of appropriate evaluation instruments
f. Determination of need for continued occupational therapy services

49. Which section of the SOAP note should include a statement about medical necessity?

a. Subjective
b. Objective
c. Assessment
d. Plan

50. Which statement is accurate regarding the use of standardized tests in the evaluation of occupational therapy clients?

a. Standardized tests provide quantitative results that can be compared to normative data.
b. Inter-rater reliability is lower for standardized tests than for non-standardized tests.
c. Modifications to the administration procedures of a standardized test will not affect the results of the test.
d. Adaptation of a standardized test from the intended client population to a different client population does not affect the validity of the results.

51. The occupational therapist (OT) completed a play assessment on a child in the home environment. She documented that the child did not have many toys but was interested in the toys that the OT brought to the home and played with them appropriately. In this situation, which factor of play is problematic?

a. The capacity to play
b. The approach to play
c. The motivation for play
d. The supportiveness of the environment

52. A COTA is providing educational materials to an elderly client who has a fifth-grade reading level and low vision. Which strategies would be beneficial to this client's health literacy?

Select the three (3) best choices.

a. Use a font size of 12.
b. Keep written instructions simple.
c. Use clear and relevant pictures.
d. Avoid oral instructions.
e. Utilize teach-back strategies.
f. Use low-contrast print.

Copyright © Mometrix Media. You have been licensed one copy of this document for personal use only. Any other reproduction or redistribution is strictly prohibited. All rights reserved.
This content is provided for test preparation purposes only and does not imply an endorsement by Mometrix of any particular political, scientific, or religious point of view.

53. Which type of wheelchair features rear wheel axles that are positioned two inches posterior to their normal position?

a. Hemiplegic
b. Reclining
c. Sports
d. Amputee

54. Which diagnosis would be MOST appropriately treated with constraint-induced movement therapy to improve upper extremity function?

a. Cerebral palsy
b. Osteoarthritis
c. Rheumatoid arthritis
d. Muscular dystrophy

55. An occupational therapist's daily note indicates that a patient is able to move and stack cones with smooth and fluid movement of the upper extremity. This is best described as an example of which motor skill?

a. Moves
b. Coordinates
c. Lifts
d. Flows

56. Which skill is both a motor skill and a process skill?

a. Initiating
b. Sequencing
c. Pacing
d. Coordinating

57. Which intervention would be contraindicated for a patient with trigger finger?

a. Fabrication of a splint
b. Repetitive gripping activities
c. Modalities to address inflammation
d. Tendon protection techniques

58. A patient with deformities of the hands due to rheumatoid arthritis is being seen for occupational therapy services in the outpatient setting. Which joint protective techniques should be taught to this patient?

Select the three (3) best choices.

a. Turn doorknobs by turning in the direction of the thumb.
b. Lift plates with the palms of both hands.
c. Hold a vegetable peeler diagonally across the palm of the hand.
d. Stir by moving the spoon in a clockwise position for a right-handed person.
e. Move objects in the kitchen by sliding them on the countertop.
f. Open a jar by using the left hand.

Copyright © Mometrix Media. You have been licensed one copy of this document for personal use only. Any other reproduction or redistribution is strictly prohibited. All rights reserved.
This content is provided for test preparation purposes only and does not imply an endorsement by Mometrix of any particular political, scientific, or religious point of view.

59. A patient is in an acute inpatient rehab setting due to a recent cerebrovascular accident. The COTA is having the patient push a ball on a table with both hands clasped on top of the ball. Which intervention is BEST described by this treatment technique?

a. Constraint-induced movement
b. Repetitive task practice
c. Bilateral upper extremity integration

60. A physician is concerned about his patient with scoliosis who is currently wheelchair bound. He feels that her current wheelchair is inadequate and is requesting that the occupational therapist (OT) assess the patient. During the evaluation, the patient indicates to the OT that the degree of her scoliotic curve has worsened in the past two years, resulting in increased levels of back pain. She is concerned that continued use of her current wheelchair will lead to more pain. After collaboration among the OT, physician and patient, the occupational therapy outcome for this patient was established as follows: "The patient will obtain an appropriate wheelchair postural support system." This is an example of which outcome category?

a. Prevention
b. Improvement
c. Enhancement

61. An early-intervention occupational therapist evaluated a 12-month-old infant with developmental delay. She noted in the evaluation that the infant currently demonstrated the developmental milestones of a 6-month-old infant. Which developmental milestones would the infant MOST likely be able to perform?

Select the three (3) best choices.

a. Voluntary suck
b. Babbling sounds
c. Commando crawl
d. Inferior pincer grasp
e. Independent sitting
f. Munching pattern

Copyright © Mometrix Media. You have been licensed one copy of this document for personal use only. Any other reproduction or redistribution is strictly prohibited. All rights reserved.
This content is provided for test preparation purposes only and does not imply an endorsement by Mometrix of any particular political, scientific, or religious point of view.

62. The COTA is teaching a parent how to facilitate in-hand manipulation skills with her 9-month old infant. Which prehension skill is MOST appropriate for this infant?

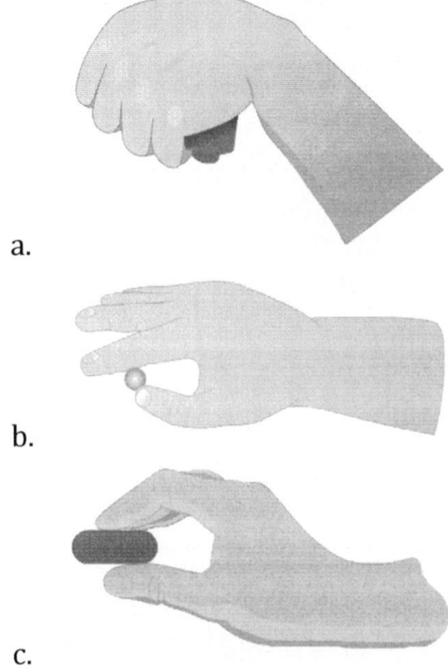

a.

b.

c.

63. The occupational therapist evaluation of a 6-year old child indicates that the child's pencil gripping technique is consistent with the developmental age of a 3-year-old. Which pencil grip is this child MOST likely to display?

a. Static tripod
b. Dynamic tripod
c. Palmar supinate

64. Which pre-academic skills would a typical 2-year-old child be able to perform?

Select the three (3) best choices.

a. Trace along a thick line.
b. Follow three-step commands.
c. Paste pieces of paper.
d. Stack nine blocks.
e. Sort by size or color.
f. Match circles, triangles, and squares.

65. A patient with a history of severe osteoporosis has thoracic pain that is typically rated as 3/10 on the pain scale, with 10 being severe. She presents to the occupational therapy (OT)_department for her scheduled outpatient OT session and reports that her thoracic pain is now 9/10 on the pain scale and seemed to start after a coughing episode. Which action would be MOST appropriate for the COTA to take?

a. Decrease the intensity of her postural exercises, and apply heat to her thoracic area.
b. Do not commence treatment, and notify the occupational therapist of the change in status.
c. Modify the treatment and focus the session on patient education instead of active exercise.

Copyright © Mometrix Media. You have been licensed one copy of this document for personal use only. Any other reproduction or redistribution is strictly prohibited. All rights reserved.
This content is provided for test preparation purposes only and does not imply an endorsement by Mometrix of any particular political, scientific, or religious point of view.

66. A patient is receiving inpatient rehabilitation services due to a recent cerebrovascular accident. During an occupational therapy session, slight movement of the patient's affected hand was observed while she was squeezing a small ball in her unaffected hand. Which Brunnstrom stage of motor recovery would correlate with this phenomenon?

a. Stage 1
b. Stage 3
c. Stage 5
d. Stage 7

67. Proper setup of a computer workstation involves which postural considerations?

a. Elbows should be flexed to 90–100 degrees.
b. Hips should be flexed to 70–80 degrees.
c. Wrists should be flexed to 45 degrees.
d. Eyes should gaze downward 45 degrees.

68. Which task progression is the BEST example of grading of endurance?

a. Progress from buttoning large coat buttons to buttoning the buttons on a blouse.
b. Progress from placing a plate in an overhead cabinet to placing a bag of flour in an overhead cabinet.
c. Progress from standing at the kitchen sink to wash the breakfast dishes to standing at the kitchen counter to prepare a complete meal.

69. Pressure areas during wrist splint fabrication can be avoided by following which guideline?

a. Splint should be three-quarters the length of the forearm.
b. Proximal and distal edges of the splint should be flared.
c. Internal and external corners should be angular.

70. Which fine motor control milestone should be achieved by 3 years of age?

a. Manipulate squeeze bottles.
b. Hold up fingers to tell age.
c. Use table utensils skillfully.

71. Which activity would be considered professional development that would meet continuing competency requirements for a COTA?

a. Occupational Safety and Health Administration (OSHA) blood-borne pathogen training
b. Corporate compliance training
c. Cardiopulmonary resuscitation training

72. Which actions would be MOST appropriate in the treatment of a stage one pressure wound?

Select the three (3) best choices.

a. Absorb exudate.
b. Relieve pressure.
c. Keep area clean.
d. Avoid shearing forces.
e. Remove eschar.
f. Maintain a moist wound bed.

Copyright © Mometrix Media. You have been licensed one copy of this document for personal use only. Any other reproduction or redistribution is strictly prohibited. All rights reserved.
This content is provided for test preparation purposes only and does not imply an endorsement by Mometrix of any particular political, scientific, or religious point of view.

73. A COTA is assisting a patient in the acute care hospital with bed mobility. The patient underwent a left posterolateral total hip replacement one day ago. Which precaution is MOST appropriate for this patient with regard to the supine position?

a. Maintain the left hip in slight adduction and internal rotation.
b. Maintain the left hip in slight abduction and neutral rotation.
c. Maintain the left hip in slight abduction and internal rotation.
d. Maintain the left hip in slight adduction and neutral rotation.

74. During the Clinical Test for Sensory Interaction in Balance (CTSIB), which condition will cause maximal instability in a patient with vestibular dysfunction?

a. Visual conflict with moving surround, moving platform
b. Eyes closed, stable surface
c. Visual conflict with moving surround, stable surface
d. Eyes open, moving surface

75. A patient with a traumatic brain injury is noted to have difficulty sorting and matching socks while folding laundry in occupational therapy. Which perceptual disorder is MOST likely responsible for this impairment?

a. Form discrimination
b. Depth perception
c. Figure-ground discrimination

76. Which statement best describes a principle of universal design?

a. The design shall utilize lower-end building supplies to make the home financially feasible to all home buyers.
b. The design shall be based on equitable use that does not disadvantage any group of users.
c. The design shall utilize customized size and space features based on the homeowner's specific needs.

77. Which technique may be utilized by the clinician when ambulating with a patient to reduce the risk of falls?

a. Guard the patient from a position that is anterolateral to the patient's body.
b. Place one hand on the gait belt and the other hand on the upper arm.
c. Move forward in step with the patient, maintaining a wide base of support.

78. A patient's home is being modified to make it wheelchair accessible. Which specifications meet the standards set by the Americans with Disabilities Act?

a. Bed height should be 26 inches from the floor.
b. Ramps should have no more than 2:12 ramp slope ratio.
c. Door width should be 38 inches at a minimum.
d. Sink height should be 32–34 inches from the floor.

79. Which intervention is an example of a lifestyle accommodation in the treatment of a child with a sensory-processing disorder?

a. Provide the child with seamless clothes with the tags removed.
b. Incorporate gradual vestibular input through play-based activities.
c. Replace fluorescent lighting with dimmer lighting options.

Copyright © Mometrix Media. You have been licensed one copy of this document for personal use only. Any other reproduction or redistribution is strictly prohibited. All rights reserved.
This content is provided for test preparation purposes only and does not imply an endorsement by Mometrix of any particular political, scientific, or religious point of view.

80. An adult who is participating in an occupational therapy group is being difficult and disrupting the group activity. Which redirection techniques are MOST appropriate in this situation?

Select the three (3) best choices.

a. Use the disruption as a teaching moment for the group.
b. Use the person's name, and ask him or her a question related to the activity.
c. Enlist the person's help by giving him or her a responsibility.
d. Enlist the help of another member of the group to serve as a mentor.
e. Use an authoritative tone of voice to refocus the participant's attention.
f. Use proximity by standing or sitting near the person.

81. Which combined shoulder motions are MOST likely to cause an anterior dislocation of the shoulder in a patient with a Bankart lesion?

a. Shoulder abduction and flexion
b. Shoulder internal rotation and abduction
c. Shoulder internal rotation and horizontal adduction
d. Shoulder external rotation and abduction

82. The following picture (with motion occurring in the direction indicated) is an example of a strengthening exercise for which muscles?

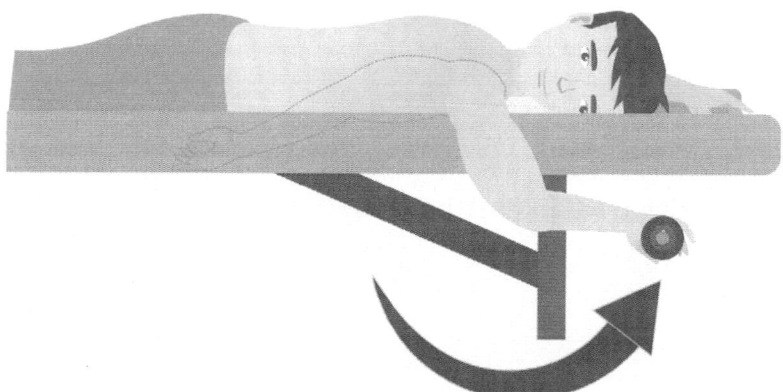

a. Subscapularis
b. Supraspinatus
c. Teres minor

83. Which statement correctly identifies the MOST appropriate technique for the mobilization of tendon adhesions?

a. The tendon should be positioned in the lengthened position; friction massage is performed perpendicular to the tendon.
b. The tendon should be positioned in the mid-range position; friction massage is performed in line with the tendon.
c. The tendon should be positioned in the shortened position; friction massage is performed in line with the tendon.
d. The tendon should be placed in a position of comfort; friction massage is performed perpendicular to the tendon.

Copyright © Mometrix Media. You have been licensed one copy of this document for personal use only. Any other reproduction or redistribution is strictly prohibited. All rights reserved.
This content is provided for test preparation purposes only and does not imply an endorsement by Mometrix of any particular political, scientific, or religious point of view.

84. A patient with a diagnosis of paraplegia was noted by the occupational therapist to have good upper extremity strength as well as good sitting balance. The COTA is tasked with instructing the patient to dress in the seated position. Which list correctly identifies the order for donning clothes from first to last?

a. Socks, shirt, undergarments, pants, shoes
b. Shirt, undergarments, pants, socks, shoes
c. Undergarments, pants, socks, shoes, shirt
d. Socks, undergarments, pants, shoes, shirt

85. A COTA is scheduled to perform transfer training with a patient who weighs 300 pounds and is 1-day s/p right TKA with WBAT on the right lower extremity. Which intervention is MOST appropriate for this patient?

a. Transfer training with assist of one person to a reclining wheelchair with elevating leg rests
b. Transfer training with assist of two people to a bariatric wheelchair with elevating leg rests
c. Transfer training with assist of one person to a bariatric wheelchair with foot rests
d. Transfer training with assist of two people to a reclining wheelchair with foot rests

86. The occupational therapy evaluation for a patient with Guillain-Barré Syndrome indicates that the patient requires total assistance for transfers. Which device is MOST appropriate to use to transfer this patient from a bed to a wheelchair?

a. Air-assistive device
b. Sliding board
c. Stand-assist lift
d. Mechanical lift

87. A patient with which level of spinal cord injury and associated ASIA impairment grade is MOST likely to require total assistance with transfers?

a. C5 ASIA A
b. C5 ASIA E
c. C7 ASIA B
d. C7 ASIA D

88. A surgeon has included continuous passive motion with a CPM machine as part of the postoperative protocol for a rotator cuff repair. During the maximum protection phase of rehabilitation, which two shoulder motions should be addressed with the CPM?

a. Elevation and internal rotation in the plane of the scapula
b. Abduction and external rotation
c. Elevation and external rotation in the plane of the scapula
d. Abduction and internal rotation

89. Which rationales BEST describe the purpose of clinical documentation? Select the three (3) best choices.

a. Communication with community resources
b. Continuity of care among rehab professionals
c. Provision of clinical information to the patient
d. Chronological record of care
e. Maintenance of exercise log
f. Reimbursement requirement

Copyright © Mometrix Media. You have been licensed one copy of this document for personal use only. Any other reproduction or redistribution is strictly prohibited. All rights reserved.
This content is provided for test preparation purposes only and does not imply an endorsement by Mometrix of any particular political, scientific, or religious point of view.

90. An individualized education plan (IEP) was written for Marissa, a seventh-grade student who has decreased fine and gross motor skills, impaired visual motor skills, distractibility issues, and impaired receptive and written language skills. As a result, she has difficulty completing assignments on time. Which IEP goal is BEST suited for Marissa?

a. Marissa will use identified accommodations and adaptations and/or assistive technology to complete her assignments within the classroom setting in the same amount of time as her classmates at least 75% of the time.
b. Occupational therapy staff will provide one-to-one instruction to Marissa in the use of a word processor to facilitate timely submission of class assignments in the same amount of time as her classmates at least 75% of the time.
c. Marissa will demonstrate improved fine motor tasks as noted by a 30% increase in her score on the School Assessment of Motor and Process Skills (AMPS).
d. Occupational therapy staff will perform skilled observation of Marissa in the classroom setting to assess her fine motor skills during educational tasks.

91. Which handling techniques should be utilized when working with a patient who exhibits upper extremity flexor hypertonicity?

Select the three (3) best choices.

a. Place your hand over the biceps on the affected upper extremity.
b. Place your hand over the triceps on the affected upper extremity.
c. Perform passive range of motion to the first or fifth digit of the affected upper extremity.
d. Perform passive range of motion to digits two, three, and four of the affected upper extremity.
e. Place your hand in the patient's affected hand from the ulnar side.
f. Place your hand in the patient's affected hand from the radial side.

92. A COTA noted that members of an occupational therapy group worked on activities side by side with an awareness of the other group members, but little interaction occurred among the group members. This scenario best describes which level of social participation?

a. Associative participation
b. Parallel participation
c. Supportive cooperative participation
d. Mature participation

93. Which statement best describes the neurodevelopmental treatment (NDT) approach?

a. NDT is based on four sequential phases related to the development of motor control: reciprocal inhibition, co-contraction, heavy work, and skill.
b. NDT utilizes mass and synergistic patterns of movement through multiple planes of motion in conjunction with faciliatory techniques.
c. NDT utilizes physical handling techniques and key points of control to support body segments and assist the patient in regaining active control.

94. A group of patients with a variety of diagnoses are playing cards in a group therapy setting. Which adaptation to card playing would be most beneficial to a patient with rheumatoid arthritis?

a. Card sorter
b. Card holder
c. Large size cards

Copyright © Mometrix Media. You have been licensed one copy of this document for personal use only. Any other reproduction or redistribution is strictly prohibited. All rights reserved.
This content is provided for test preparation purposes only and does not imply an endorsement by Mometrix of any particular political, scientific, or religious point of view.

95. Which anatomical sites are MOST likely to be potential pressure points when using a wrist immobilization splint?

Select the three (3) best choices.

a. Radial styloid
b. Base of the first proximal phalange
c. Ulnar styloid
d. Thumb web space
e. Lateral epicondyle
f. Head of the first metacarpal

96. A patient with a diagnosis of a crush injury to the hand has significant subacute edema. Which modality is MOST appropriate to treat the edema?

a. Contrast bath
b. Cold pack
c. Transcutaneous electrical nerve stimulation (TENS) unit

97. Which medical conditions would be a contraindication for the use of thermotherapy?

a. Pregnancy
b. Cardiac insufficiency
c. Thrombophlebitis

98. Which type of electrical stimulation is MOST appropriate to improve motor control in a patient who has had a stroke?

a. Transcutaneous electrical nerve stimulation
b. Neuromuscular electrical stimulation
c. Direct current electrical muscle stimulation

99. Which intervention is the MOST effective treatment for hypertrophic scarring?

a. Passive stretch
b. Massage
c. Positioning
d. Compression

100. A COTA is using electrical stimulation to promote wound healing on a patient, utilizing a saline-soaked gauze directly in the wound, covered by a single-use disposable electrode. Which statement is true with regard to the setup for this type of treatment?

a. A large dispersive pad of the same polarity should be placed on the outer edge of the wound.
b. A large dispersive pad of the opposite polarity should be placed on the outer edge of the wound.
c. A large dispersive pad of the opposite polarity should be placed several inches away from the wound.
d. A large dispersive pad of the same polarity should be placed several inches away from the wound.

101. Which technique is MOST appropriate to promote swallowing in a 4-year-old child?

a. Position the child in a semi-reclined position.
b. Utilize verbal cues to facilitate swallowing.
c. Encourage the child to suck on an ice pop.

Copyright © Mometrix Media. You have been licensed one copy of this document for personal use only. Any other reproduction or redistribution is strictly prohibited. All rights reserved.
This content is provided for test preparation purposes only and does not imply an endorsement by Mometrix of any particular political, scientific, or religious point of view.

102. Which activity is an example of relational play?

a. Making a pretend meal
b. Stacking blocks
c. Banging a rattle

103. A COTA is working with a child who has poor upper extremity strength and minimal hand movement. Which assistive technology switch would be MOST appropriate for this child to use?

a. Button switch
b. Grasp switch
c. Ribbon switch
d. Plate switch

104. Which splint is MOST appropriate for a patient with an ulnar nerve injury?

a. Anti-claw
b. Wrist cock-up
c. Thumb spica

105. Which mental function is most challenged during meal preparation tasks?

a. Thought
b. Experience of self and time
c. Attention
d. Emotion

106. Which activity of daily living is MOST likely to require adaptations for a patient with a recent posterolateral total hip replacement who is on hip precautions?

a. Donning socks and shoes
b. Donning bra and shirt
c. Washing dishes
d. Brushing teeth

107. A school administrative team has requested input from the occupational therapist and COTA regarding the purchase of new playground equipment that would be appropriate for children with physical disabilities. This is an example of which intervention approach?

a. Training
b. Consultation
c. Advocacy
d. Prevention

108. Which hand position is characterized by flexion of the MCP joints, full extension of the IP joints, and 10–30 degrees of wrist extension?

a. Safe
b. Functional
c. Resting

Copyright © Mometrix Media. You have been licensed one copy of this document for personal use only. Any other reproduction or redistribution is strictly prohibited. All rights reserved.
This content is provided for test preparation purposes only and does not imply an endorsement by Mometrix of any particular political, scientific, or religious point of view.

109. The occupational therapy evaluation indicates that a patient displays uncontrolled, purposeless, jerking movements. Which movement pattern BEST describes this patient's movement disorder?

a. Athetoid
b. Ballism
c. Choreiform

110. A patient is being instructed in the concept of neutral position during simulated lifting activities. Which upper extremity positions are characteristic of the neutral position?

Select the three (3) best choices.

a. Shoulders are abducted 20 degrees.
b. Shoulders are positioned at one's sides.
c. Elbows are flexed 90 degrees.
d. Elbows are flexed 45 degrees.
e. Forearms are fully supinated.
f. Forearms are in neutral position.

111. Which action is MOST appropriate for the treating COTA to perform for a patient who is having a seizure?

a. Gently hold the person down to prevent further injury.
b. Clear the immediate area of objects that could cause further injury.
c. Place a tongue depressor in the person's mouth to prevent biting of the tongue.

112. Which intervention is MOST appropriate as part of a desensitization program after a partial finger amputation?

a. Stimulation of the fingertip with a variety of textures
b. Submersion of the finger in a container of lukewarm water
c. Passive range of motion of the involved finger

113. Injury to which nerve would result in the inability to flex the thumb tip and index fingertip to the palm of the hand?

a. Radial
b. Ulnar
c. Median

114. Which injury is another name for a fracture of the neck of the fourth or fifth metacarpal?

a. Bennett fracture
b. Boxer's fracture
c. Colles' fracture
d. Smith fracture

115. Which finger deformity is caused by damage to the extensor tendon mechanism, resulting in a flexion contracture of the distal interphalangeal (DIP) joint?

a. Boutonniére deformity
b. Dupuytren contracture
c. Mallet finger

Copyright © Mometrix Media. You have been licensed one copy of this document for personal use only. Any other reproduction or redistribution is strictly prohibited. All rights reserved.
This content is provided for test preparation purposes only and does not imply an endorsement by Mometrix of any particular political, scientific, or religious point of view.

116. Which handling characteristic should occur when low-temperature thermoplastics have been heated to the proper molding temperature?

a. Rigidity
b. Durability
c. Elasticity

117. Which condition would be the MOST appropriate indication for treatment with ultrasound?

a. Subacute inflammation
b. Edema
c. Spasticity

118. Which type of fracture is BEST described as a bone fragment that is pulled off the bone by a ligament or tendon?

a. Stress
b. Greenstick
c. Pathological
d. Avulsion

119. Which activities are appropriate interventions to reduce the risk of a deep vein thrombosis after a total knee replacement surgery?

Select the three (3) best choices.

a. Dangle the involved lower extremity when sitting.
b. Encourage seated exercises instead of standing exercises.
c. Use a pneumatic compression device when in bed.
d. Avoid walking for the first 48 hours after surgery.
e. Perform ankle pumping exercises.
f. Wear compression stockings.

120. According to Part B of the Individuals with Disabilities Education Improvement Act (IDEA), what is the ideal educational setting for individuals with a disability?

a. Self-contained classroom in public school environment
b. Private tutors in the home environment
c. Least restrictive environment

121. The occupational therapist has completed a workplace assessment and recommended engineering controls. Which change is an example of an engineering control?

a. Mandatory wearing of earplugs
b. Mandatory use of a pneumatic lifting device
c. Mandatory work breaks every two hours

122. The physician has recommended an AFO for a patient with foot drop due to a stroke. The patient has a history of poorly controlled lower extremity edema. Which type of AFO would be MOST appropriate for this patient?

a. Metal, double-upright AFO
b. Plastic, custom-hinged ankle AFO
c. Plastic, prefabricated solid-ankle AFO

Copyright © Mometrix Media. You have been licensed one copy of this document for personal use only. Any other reproduction or redistribution is strictly prohibited. All rights reserved.
This content is provided for test preparation purposes only and does not imply an endorsement by Mometrix of any particular political, scientific, or religious point of view.

123. Which activities are examples of areas of occupation?

Select the three (3) best choices.

a. Play
b. Leisure
c. Habits
d. Routines
e. Social participation
f. Rituals

124. Which carpal bone lies within the anatomical snuffbox of the hand?

a. Trapezoid
b. Trapezium
c. Capitate
d. Scaphoid

125. Which modalities may be utilized in the treatment of an open wound?

Select the three (3) best choices.

a. Paraffin bath
b. Electrical stimulation
c. Fluidotherapy
d. Whirlpool
e. Ultrasound
f. Cold pack

126. Which activities are instrumental activities of daily living?

Select the three (3) best choices.

a. Functional mobility
b. Community mobility
c. Financial management
d. Toileting
e. Eating
f. Meal preparation

127. A COTA is using a cleaning chemical to scrub the occupational therapy kitchen counter and not sure if she should wear person protective equipment while using it. Where is the MOST appropriate place to look for this information?

a. Infection control policy
b. Material safety data sheet
c. Universal precautions guidelines

128. Which action is an example of a movement function associated with the activity of brushing one's teeth?

a. Ability to feel the water and toothbrush in the mouth
b. Ability to sequence movement of the brush to different locations in the mouth
c. Ability to open the mouth, close the mouth, and swallow

Copyright © Mometrix Media. You have been licensed one copy of this document for personal use only. Any other reproduction or redistribution is strictly prohibited. All rights reserved.
This content is provided for test preparation purposes only and does not imply an endorsement by Mometrix of any particular political, scientific, or religious point of view.

129. Which muscle would be affected by an injury to the dorsal scapular nerve?

a. Trapezius
b. Levator scapula
c. Serratus anterior
d. Pectoralis minor

130. Which mental functions are examples of higher-level cognitive functions?

Select the three (3) best choices.

a. Visual discrimination
b. Logical thought
c. Concentration
d. Judgement
e. Praxis
f. Insight

131. The occupational therapy home health evaluation indicates that a patient's desired outcome is to be able to attend Sunday church services on a regular basis. This is BEST described as an example of which type of outcome?

a. Participation
b. Prevention
c. Quality of life
d. Adaptation

132. Which body part will MOST likely require splinting in a child with a diagnosis of camptodactyly?

a. Wrist
b. Elbow
c. Thumb
d. Little finger

133. Which statements are true regarding norm-referenced standardized measurement instruments?

Select the three (3) best choices.

a. Requires diagnostics skills
b. Depends on task analysis
c. Utilizes cut-off scores
d. Maximizes differences among individuals
e. Is sensitive to the effects of therapy
f. Evaluates individual performance against a group

134. Which standardized test is a criterion-referenced test that provides a uniform system measurement for disability and is frequently used in the inpatient rehabilitation setting?

a. The Functional Independence Measure
b. The Canadian Occupational Performance Measure
c. The Melville-Nelson Self-Care Assessment

Copyright © Mometrix Media. You have been licensed one copy of this document for personal use only. Any other reproduction or redistribution is strictly prohibited. All rights reserved.
This content is provided for test preparation purposes only and does not imply an endorsement by Mometrix of any particular political, scientific, or religious point of view.

135. A community hospital is developing a series of community health interventions for the senior citizens in the community. An administrator has asked the rehabilitation staff to develop an aquatic exercise class as part of the program. An aquatic exercise program would fall into which level of prevention programming?

a. Primary
b. Secondary
c. Tertiary

136. A COTA is seeing a home health patient for a 4:00 p.m. treatment session. The patient is 4 days status-post a right total hip replacement. During the visit, the patient mentions that her right calf has been hurting. The COTA notices that the calf is warm and tender to touch, discolored, and swollen. Which action is MOST appropriate in this situation?

a. Discontinue the occupational therapy session, and advise the patient to call the doctor in the morning.
b. Discontinue the occupational therapy session, and contact the evaluating occupational therapist.
c. Modify the treatment session to avoid any activities that aggravate the pain.
d. Modify the treatment session to seated exercises only, and document the rationale.

137. Which level of dysphagia diet would include finely chopped meats?

a. Level I
b. Level II
c. Level III
d. Level IV

138. Which exercises are most appropriate to promote the oral stage of swallowing?

Select the three (3) best choices.

a. Tongue base retraction exercises
b. Shaker exercises
c. Jaw range of motion exercises
d. Lip resistive exercises
e. Pitch exercises
f. Tongue range of motion exercises

139. Which balance assessment tool utilizes a self-perception scale?

a. Timed Up and Go
b. Dynamic Gait Index
c. Berg Balance Scale
d. Falls Efficacy Scale

140. Which health care providers are MOST likely to work together as a collaborative team in a mental health practice?

Select the three (3) best choices.

a. Psychiatrist
b. Social worker
c. Occupational therapist
d. Physical therapist
e. Speech therapist
f. Emergency room physician

Copyright © Mometrix Media. You have been licensed one copy of this document for personal use only. Any other reproduction or redistribution is strictly prohibited. All rights reserved.
This content is provided for test preparation purposes only and does not imply an endorsement by Mometrix of any particular political, scientific, or religious point of view.

141. Which statement is true regarding the use of a Coban pressure wrap in the treatment of edema of the hand?

a. Begin wrapping of each finger from the distal aspect to the proximal aspect.
b. Avoid active exercise while the wrap is in place.
c. Pull the wrap as tight as possible to maximize edema reduction.

142. A patient with a transhumeral amputation is being trained to control the mechanical elbow of the prosthesis. Which motions of the scapula and shoulder are used to flex the mechanical elbow?

a. Scapular abduction and shoulder abduction
b. Scapular abduction and shoulder flexion
c. Scapular adduction and shoulder abduction
d. Scapular adduction and shoulder flexion

143. Which age-related skeletal system concern is MOST likely to limit the physical activity of a middle-age adult?

a. Osteoporosis
b. Osteoarthritis
c. Back pain
d. Scoliosis

144. A COTA is having a patient with a diagnosis of a recent cerebrovascular accident locate and name specific utensils through touch while washing them in soapy water. Which condition is MOST appropriately treated through this activity?

a. Astereognosis
b. Visual agnosia
c. Apraxia

145. A COTA is instructing a patient in motor strategies for balance control. Which strategy is MOST appropriate for the patient to utilize during small perturbations?

a. Hip strategy
b. Ankle strategy
c. Stepping strategy

146. A patient is 3 weeks status-post a total shoulder arthroplasty. Which activities are contraindicated for this patient?

Select the three (3) best choices.

a. Reaching behind the back with the involved arm
b. Lifting 8 pounds with the involved arm
c. Writing with elbow at waist level with the involved arm
d. Pushing up through the involved arm to get out of a chair.
e. Light isometric exercise of the deltoid and scapulothoracic muscles of the involved arm
f. Passive range of motion up to 30 degrees of external rotation of the involved arm

Copyright © Mometrix Media. You have been licensed one copy of this document for personal use only. Any other reproduction or redistribution is strictly prohibited. All rights reserved.
This content is provided for test preparation purposes only and does not imply an endorsement by Mometrix of any particular political, scientific, or religious point of view.

147. A patient has recently undergone a PIP arthroplasty to correct a swan-neck deformity and has been referred to an occupational therapist for static digital splinting. Which position should be incorporated into the splint?

a. Neutral PIP and DIP position
b. 10–30 degrees of PIP flexion and full DIP extension
c. 45–55 degrees of PIP flexion and full DIP flexion
d. Neutral PIP position and full DIP flexion

148. A COTA is working with a patient who demonstrates poor tolerance to prolonged muscle activity. While styling her hair, the patient must lower her arms several times to rest. Which intervention BEST describes proper exercise grading for this patient?

a. Perform exercises with low repetitions and increasing amounts of resistance.
b. Perform exercises with increasing amounts of resistance while shortening the time period.
c. Perform exercises with low resistance and increase the number of repetitions and/or time period.

149. A COTA is monitoring the vital signs of a patient with a history of cardiopulmonary dysfunction. Which change in vital signs during activity would warrant discontinuation of the activity and notification of the occupational therapist?

a. A drop in heartrate from 80 beats/minute at rest to 70 beats/minute with activity
b. An increase in heart rate from 80 beats/minute at rest to 100 beats/minute with activity
c. An increase in systolic blood pressure from 135 mm Hg at rest to 150 mm Hg with activity
d. An increase in diastolic blood pressure from 80 mm Hg at rest to 85 mm Hg with activity

150. A child with weakness of the lumbrical muscles has poor handwriting. Which progression best describes grading of an activity that is appropriate for this child?

a. Progress from tracing large letters to tracing small letters using a pencil.
b. Progress from simulated writing activities with tongs to the use of smaller writing utensils.
c. Progress from printing letters to writing the letters in cursive.

151. Which activities BEST exemplify scholarly activities relative to evidence-based practice in occupational therapy?

Select the three (3) best choices.

a. Attendance at the annual AOTA conference
b. Attendance at interdisciplinary patient rounds
c. Participation in a clinical research study of stroke patients
d. Participation in annual infection control training
e. Review of articles in *The American Journal of Occupational Therapy*
f. Review of blog postings on AOTA's website.

152. Which factors should be considered when planning an intervention to facilitate leisure activities?

Select the three (3) best choices.

a. Self-care skills
b. Freedom of choice
c. Suspension of reality
d. Sense of competence
e. Job demands
f. Intrinsic satisfaction

Copyright © Mometrix Media. You have been licensed one copy of this document for personal use only. Any other reproduction or redistribution is strictly prohibited. All rights reserved.
This content is provided for test preparation purposes only and does not imply an endorsement by Mometrix of any particular political, scientific, or religious point of view.

153. A patient is referred to an occupational therapist for treatment of hand pain. Which diagnosis is MOST appropriately treated by a paraffin bath?

a. An acute crush injury
b. Recent trigger finger release
c. Rheumatoid arthritis

154. Which play activity may be contraindicated in a child with Downs syndrome?

a. Tumbling
b. Playing catch
c. Kicking a ball

155. A COTA is treating a patient with a spinal cord injury that occurred 1 month ago. The patient is noted to have swelling, warmth, and decreased range of motion at the elbow. The COTA should be concerned about the possibility of which condition?

a. Osteoporosis
b. Heterotopic ossification
c. Spasticity
d. Autonomic dysreflexia

156. Which instructions are appropriate to provide to a patient who is learning to independently ascend a curb in a wheelchair?

a. Position the chair close to and facing the curb, then perform a partial wheelie to elevate the caster wheels onto the upper surface of the curb.
b. Position the rear wheels so they contact the bottom step, elevate the caster wheels, then ascend the curb backward.
c. Position the chair close to and facing the curb, then lower the anti-tip bars to prevent the wheelchair from tipping over while ascending the curb.

157. A patient in the intensive care unit is on a respirator and unable to verbalize his needs. Which communication device is MOST appropriate in this situation?

a. Speech-generating device
b. Virtual keyboard with a pointing system
c. Low-technology communication board

158. A patient with low vision is having difficulty seeing his plate on the table. Which strategy could the COTA utilize to make it easier for the patient to see the plate?

a. Use a light-colored plate with a dark border.
b. Place a solid-colored plate on a checkered tablecloth.
c. Place a dark-colored plate on a tablecloth of similar color.

159. Which condition would MOST likely benefit from the use of a strap connecting the two leg rests instead of heel loops on a manual wheelchair?

a. Unilateral transfemoral amputation
b. Unilateral transtibial amputation
c. L4 ASIA A spinal cord injury
d. C3 ASIA B spinal cord injury

Copyright © Mometrix Media. You have been licensed one copy of this document for personal use only. Any other reproduction or redistribution is strictly prohibited. All rights reserved.
This content is provided for test preparation purposes only and does not imply an endorsement by Mometrix of any particular political, scientific, or religious point of view.

160. Which adverse effect would be associated with a wheelchair seat width that is too wide for a patient?

a. Difficulty with sit-to-stand transfers
b. Excessive pressure to the greater trochanters
c. Inability to position the knees beneath a table

161. A COTA is teaching a patient with hemiplegia from a recent CVA how to modify the task method to perform her activities of daily living. Which examples BEST describe modifications to the task method?

Select the three (3) best choices.

a. Install a grab bar in the shower.
b. Cut vegetables on a cutting board with aluminum nails.
c. Sponge bathe at sink level.
d. Use a button hook to button shirts.
e. Dress the affected side first.
f. Tie shoes with the one-handed approach.

162. A COTA is working to improve functional strength in a patient's dominant hand. Which activity BEST describes grading of a baking activity to promote improved functional strength in the upper extremity?

a. Progress from stirring while seated to stirring while standing
b. Progress from stirring with a regular spoon to a spoon with a built-up handle
c. Progress from stirring by hand to stirring with an electric mixer
d. Progress from stirring liquids to stirring cookie batter

163. A patient with weakness of the supraspinatus muscle is performing resistive strengthening activities in standing. Which substitution pattern will MOST likely be demonstrated by this patient?

a. Ipsilateral trunk flexion
b. Ipsilateral scapular elevation
c. Ipsilateral shoulder external rotation
d. Ipsilateral shoulder internal rotation

164. Which vehicle adaptations and equipment would be MOST appropriate for an amputee with a history of multiple-level cervical fusion surgery whose primary mode of mobility is ambulation with a right transtibial prosthesis and a walker?

Select the three (3) best choices.

a. Back-up mirror
b. Wide-angle mirrors
c. Foot pedal extension
d. Hand controls
e. Wheelchair lift
f. Transfer board

Copyright © Mometrix Media. You have been licensed one copy of this document for personal use only. Any other reproduction or redistribution is strictly prohibited. All rights reserved.
This content is provided for test preparation purposes only and does not imply an endorsement by Mometrix of any particular political, scientific, or religious point of view.

165. A patient in an inpatient rehabilitation center is receiving occupational therapy services after a cerebrovascular accident. Which methods of grading are the MOST appropriate progressions of functional tasks?

Select the three (3) best choices.

a. Increasing the number of steps in an activity
b. Decreasing the number of steps in an activity
c. Decreasing the frequency of verbal cues
d. Increasing the frequency of verbal cues
e. Increasing the level of physical assistance
f. Decreasing the level of physical assistance

166. Which behavioral intervention strategies are MOST appropriate when working with an impulsive patient?

Select the three (3) best choices.

a. Provide written instructions in a step-by-step format.
b. Allow the patient to choose between among activity options.
c. Utilize a group setting approach.
d. Provide a non-distracting environment.
e. Provide verbal directions slowly.
f. Avoid repetitive tasks.

167. An occupational therapy plan of care for the treatment of a cerebral vascular accident to the left cerebral hemisphere would MOST likely include activities to address which deficits?

Select the three (3) best choices.

a. Left visual field cuts
b. Language
c. Spatial orientation
d. Time concepts
e. Analytical thinking
f. Impulsivity

168. A patient is being instructed in wheelchair mobility as part of occupational therapy treatment in an inpatient rehabilitation facility. Which manual wheelchair features would be most beneficial for a patient with a recent right-sided cerebrovascular accident, resulting in a flaccid upper extremity and spastic paralysis of the lower extremity, who also has a history of a right transfemoral amputation for which he wears a prosthesis during the day?

Select the three (3) best choices.

a. Elevating leg rests
b. Light weight
c. Brake extender
d. Quick-release wheels
e. One-arm drive
f. Projection hand rims

Copyright © Mometrix Media. You have been licensed one copy of this document for personal use only. Any other reproduction or redistribution is strictly prohibited. All rights reserved.
This content is provided for test preparation purposes only and does not imply an endorsement by Mometrix of any particular political, scientific, or religious point of view.

169. Which verbal instructions would be MOST appropriate when teaching pursed lip breathing to a client with chronic obstructive pulmonary disease (COPD)?

a. Exhale through the nose, allowing the nostrils to flare.
b. Purse your lips in the whistling position, then inhale.
c. Exhale slowly to allow exhalation to take twice as long as inhalation.

170. The COTA is instructing a patient with chronic obstructive pulmonary disease (COPD) in dyspnea control postures to utilize while grocery shopping with her husband. Which example BEST describes an appropriate dyspnea control posture?

a. Use a front-wheeled walker, pushing up through your arms to obtain an erect posture.
b. Use a shopping cart, and lean your body forward with the forearms propped on the shopping cart.
c. Use bilateral axillary crutches, leaning forward to weight bear through the axillae on the pads of the crutches.
d. Use bilateral forearm crutches, straighten the elbows, and raise the chest toward the ceiling.

171. Which principles are the MOST important considerations for client-centered groups? Select the three (3) best choices.

a. Utilize scholarly research to determine the best frame of reference for the group activity.
b. Select a frame of reference for the group activity based on the clients' input.
c. Focus on the person-environment-occupation relationship.
d. Develop a therapeutic relationship with the group members through therapeutic use of self.
e. Create structured group activities that can be generalized to all group members.
f. Guide the group members to promote change in their behavior.

172. A patient is in the maximum protection phase of rehabilitation after a total elbow arthroplasty. Which statements accurately reflect guidelines for this phase of rehabilitation for this diagnosis?

Select the three (3) best choices.

a. Perform AROM exercises to maximize end-range elbow flexion.
b. Strengthen the shoulder utilizing cuff weights placed distal to the elbow.
c. Perform AROM exercises to the shoulder, wrist, and hand.
d. Strengthen the elbow through resisted isometric exercises.
e. Perform self-assisted elbow flexion and extension exercises.
f. Perform self-assisted forearm pronation and supination with the elbow partially flexed.

Copyright © Mometrix Media. You have been licensed one copy of this document for personal use only. Any other reproduction or redistribution is strictly prohibited. All rights reserved.
This content is provided for test preparation purposes only and does not imply an endorsement by Mometrix of any particular political, scientific, or religious point of view.

173. A patient with severe rheumatoid arthritis, including a significant decrease in grip strength and a severe ulnar drift, would benefit most from which adaptive utensil?

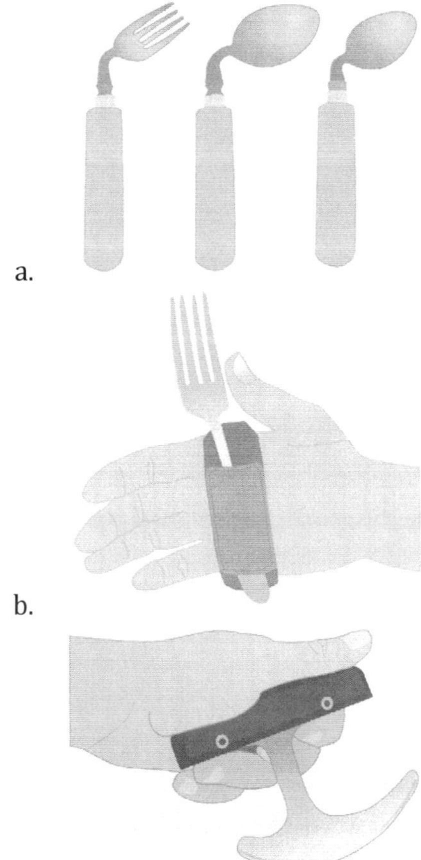

a.

b.

c.

174. A patient with Alzheimer's disease is noted to choke on thin liquids. Which strategy would be MOST appropriate to teach this patient and his caregiver?

a. Use of a flow-control cup
b. Use of a cup with a weighted bottom
c. Use of a two-handled cup

175. A COTA is working on balance with a patient and plans to make the balance activity more challenging by reducing the somatosensory cues. Which balance activity progressions are MOST appropriate in this scenario?

Select the three (3) best choices.

a. Have the patient close his or her eyes.
b. Have the patient wear prism glasses.
c. Change the supporting surface from the firm ground to a foam cushion.
d. Narrow the base of support.
e. Have the patient stand on an incline board.
f. Include activities in which the patient moves the eyes and head together.

Copyright © Mometrix Media. You have been licensed one copy of this document for personal use only. Any other reproduction or redistribution is strictly prohibited. All rights reserved.
This content is provided for test preparation purposes only and does not imply an endorsement by Mometrix of any particular political, scientific, or religious point of view.

176. Which exercise is a closed-chain strengthening exercise?

a. Bicep curls with free weights
b. Lateral pulldown on resistive equipment
c. Wall push-ups
d. Grip strengthening with a spring-loader exerciser

177. Which modality is MOST appropriate for pain control post-operatively in the days immediately following a capsulotomy surgery?

a. Transcutaneous electrical nerve stimulation (TENS)
b. Neuromuscular electrical stimulation (NMES)
c. Hydrocollator packs
d. Continuous ultrasound

178. Which orthosis would be MOST appropriate to reduce hip adductor spasticity and to improve sitting balance in a child with cerebral palsy?

a. Hip-knee-ankle-foot orthosis (HKAFO)
b. Wilmington brace
c. Standing, walking, and sitting hip (SWASH) orthosis
d. Milwaukee brace

179. Which area of attention can be treated by utilizing the Stroop effect?

a. Focused
b. Sustained
c. Selective
d. Alternating

180. A Velcro buddy splint can be MOST appropriately used to promote which action?

a. Movement of a stiff finger
b. Limitation of full range of motion of a postsurgical finger
c. Immobilization after a flexor tendon repair in a finger

181. A job analysis was performed on an injured worker whose job title is data entry clerk. Which adjustments would be MOST appropriate for this worker as part of his or her return to work program?

Select the three (3) best choices.

a. Begin at a 4-hour/day schedule, and slowly increase to an 8-hour/day schedule.
b. Provide ergonomic changes to the workstation.
c. Provide work breaks in accordance with state law.
d. Start with a reduced productivity requirement, and gradually increase to the prior level.
e. Limit prolonged standing to 15-minute intervals.
f. Require a second person to assist with lifting more than 50 pounds.

Copyright © Mometrix Media. You have been licensed one copy of this document for personal use only. Any other reproduction or redistribution is strictly prohibited. All rights reserved.
This content is provided for test preparation purposes only and does not imply an endorsement by Mometrix of any particular political, scientific, or religious point of view.

182. A 40-year-old female with multiple sclerosis is independent in all aspects of self-care and home mobility as long as she paces her activities to avoid fatigue. Which type of medical equipment would be MOST appropriate to allow her to achieve independent functional mobility at the community level?

a. Rolling walker
b. Manual wheelchair
c. Motorized scooter
d. Rollator

183. Which areas on the body would be contraindications for treatment with electrical stimulation?

Select the three (3) best choices.

a. The anterior cervical region
b. A cancerous area
c. An open wound
d. Fragile skin
e. An osteomyelitic area
f. An area of complex regional pain

184. Which conditions of the affected area would be considered contraindications for continuous passive motion (CPM) of the joint?

Select the three (3) best choices.

a. Osteoarthritis
b. Unstable fractures
c. Recent orthopedic surgery
d. Spasticity
e. Postsurgical wound
f. Uncontrolled infection

185. Which conditions are contraindications for the use of an intermittent compression pump?

Select the three (3) best choices.

a. Acute local dermatologic infection
b. Venous edema
c. Venous leg ulcer
d. Acute pulmonary edema
e. Lymphedema
f. Congestive heart failure

186. Which vital sign information is utilized when determining the inflation pressure of the intermittent compression pump?

a. Systolic blood pressure
b. Diastolic blood pressure
c. Resting heart rate
d. Maximum heart rate

Copyright © Mometrix Media. You have been licensed one copy of this document for personal use only. Any other reproduction or redistribution is strictly prohibited. All rights reserved.
This content is provided for test preparation purposes only and does not imply an endorsement by Mometrix of any particular political, scientific, or religious point of view.

187. Which pre-gait activities are MOST appropriate for a patient who exhibits pusher syndrome?

a. Passively move the patient into the desired position, and provide verbal cues to maintain the position.
b. Work on midline orientation in standing with the use of a mirror to provide feedback.
c. Raise the height of the assistive device so the patient has to bear weight on the involved side.

188. When grading meal preparation activities, which is the BEST example of a beginning-level meal preparation activity?

a. Microwaving a bag of popcorn
b. Boiling a hot dog
c. Preparing a lunchmeat and crackers snack

189. Which change to an activity BEST describes grading of social context?

a. Add a level of competition to the activity.
b. Add a level of frustration to the activity.
c. Increase the memory demands of the activity.
d. Require the patient to initiate the activity.

190. Which strategies to foster good group dynamics are MOST appropriate when dealing with school-age students in a group setting?

Select the three (3) best choices.

a. Predetermine specific behavioral rules.
b. Set a time-out chair in the hallway for poorly behaved students.
c. Format the activity as a game.
d. Make each student earn the privilege of group participation.
e. Address all levels of behavioral issues equally.
f. Use a behavioral modification program to reward positive behavior.

191. Which prosthetic knee is MOST appropriate for a patient with a transtibial amputation and cognitive deficits?

a. Weight-activated knee
b. Microprocessor knee
c. Locking knee

192. Which type of prosthetic suspension requires the patient to don a thin sock on the residual limb then pull the sock through a valve after donning the prosthetic socket?

a. Total suction
b. Supracondylar cuff
c. Thigh corset
d. Liner with locking pin

Copyright © Mometrix Media. You have been licensed one copy of this document for personal use only. Any other reproduction or redistribution is strictly prohibited. All rights reserved.
This content is provided for test preparation purposes only and does not imply an endorsement by Mometrix of any particular political, scientific, or religious point of view.

193. A COTA is educating a patient in residual limb hygiene after the surgical site has fully healed. Which instructions are MOST appropriate to provide to this patient?

Select the three (3) best choices.

a. Use rubbing alcohol to prevent infection.
b. Wash the limb in warm water.
c. Allow the limb to air dry.
d. Use lotion on the limb after bathing.
e. Use a long-handled mirror to inspect the skin integrity.
f. Bathe in the evening.

194. Which treatments are MOST appropriate to control edema in the residual limb of a patient with a transtibial amputation?

Select the three (3) best choices.

a. Use of a removable rigid dressing
b. Placement of a pillow under the knee
c. Residual limb-wrapping techniques
d. Transcutaneous electrical nerve stimulation (TENS)
e. Friction massage techniques
f. Use of a residual limb shrinker

195. Which type of exercise is MOST appropriate to promote postural stability?

a. Multiple-angle isometrics
b. Slow reversal hold
c. Rhythmic initiation
d. Rhythmic stabilization

196. Which limitations related to swallowing would be MOST appropriately treated with the Mendelsohn maneuver?

Select the three (3) best choices.

a. Reduced pharyngeal contraction
b. Reduced closure at the laryngeal entrance
c. Reduced laryngeal excursion
d. Limited cricopharyngeal opening
e. Slow pharyngeal transit
f. Reduced base of tongue movement

197. Which recommendations are appropriate guidelines for computer station ergonomics.

Select the three (3) best choices.

a. Place the computer screen 10 inches from the eyes.
b. Place the computer screen 20 inches from the eyes.
c. Position the monitor so the top border of the screen is slightly above eye level.
d. Position the monitor so the top border of the screen is slightly below eye level.
e. Maintain shoulders in a relaxed position at the side of the body.
f. Maintain shoulders in approximately 30 degrees of abduction.

Copyright © Mometrix Media. You have been licensed one copy of this document for personal use only. Any other reproduction or redistribution is strictly prohibited. All rights reserved.
This content is provided for test preparation purposes only and does not imply an endorsement by Mometrix of any particular political, scientific, or religious point of view.

198. Which position of the wrist is MOST appropriate to stretch the wrist extensors?

a. Flexion and ulnar deviation
b. Flexion and radial deviation
c. Extension and ulnar deviation
d. Extension and radial deviation

199. A patient with left hemiparesis has grossly poor + strength of the shoulder musculature. Which pieces of equipment would be MOST appropriate for this patient to utilize for exercise at this stage in rehabilitation?

Select the three (3) best choices.

a. Cable column
b. TheraBand
c. Cuff weights
d. Powder board
e. Suspension sling
f. Skateboard

200. A patient with complex regional pain syndrome is being seen for occupational therapy services. The plan of care includes desensitization activities due to tactile hyperesthesia and allodynia. Which desensitization tool would be MOST appropriate to use in the early stage of desensitization?

a. Constant pressure
b. Friction massage
c. Fluidotherapy

Copyright © Mometrix Media. You have been licensed one copy of this document for personal use only. Any other reproduction or redistribution is strictly prohibited. All rights reserved.
This content is provided for test preparation purposes only and does not imply an endorsement by Mometrix of any particular political, scientific, or religious point of view.

Answer Key and Explanations

1. C: According to Principle 1, the disclosure of any criminal, legal, or other disciplinary matters must occur within 60 days of occurrence.

2. B, D, E: Secondary rotator cuff impingement is caused by glenohumeral instability that leads to a reduction in the subacromial space. This reduced subacromial space causes anatomical crowding and can impinge the rotator cuff tendons. This glenohumeral instability is due to muscular imbalance and weakness of the scapular stabilizers. Thus, the muscles requiring strengthening would be the scapular stabilizers: lower trapezius, rhomboid major, and serratus anterior. The rotator cuff muscles (teres minor, infraspinatus, and supraspinatus) would not be addressed in the initial home exercise program.

3. B, C, D: While seated in a wheelchair, the areas most likely to develop pressure injuries are the olecranon process, the ischial tuberosity, and the vertebral spinous process. The olecranon process is subject to pressure from the armrests of the wheelchair. The ischial tuberosity is subject to pressure from the seat. The vertebral spinous process is subject to pressure from the backrest. The lateral malleolus would not be subject to pressure in the seated position but would be subject to pressure in the side-lying position on the lowermost lower extremity or possibly in the supine position if the lower extremity is externally rotated. The head of the fibula would not be subject to pressure in the seated position but could be subject to pressure in the supine position. The lateral condyle of the femur would not be subject to pressure in the seated position but could be subject to pressure in the side-lying position (lowermost lower extremity).

4. A: An MRSA infection utilizes contact isolation precautions. The required personal protective equipment for contact isolation consists of gloves and a gown. A mask would be required for droplet or airborne isolation. A respirator would be utilized for a patient who has both airborne and contact precautions.

5. B: During the active inflammatory period of rheumatoid arthritis, treatments should include joint protection, pain reduction, minimizing muscle atrophy, and maintaining available motion. Exercises during this period should include passive or active-assistive range of motion in pain-free ranges and gentle isometrics in pain-free positions. Joints should not be stressed by resistive exercise or stretching. Exercise performance should occur multiple times during the day for short durations of time.

6. C: Children with autism have difficulty processing auditory information and require simple directions. Therefore, the least effective form of communication with the child would be to provide a two-step command. The use of combined verbal and visual information would be beneficial when communicating with a child with autism. Likewise, addressing the child to get the child's attention before providing instruction would also be effective.

7. D: This answer indicates that both a change in medical status and function occurred due to a fall. The statement that the patient requires moderate assistance does not provide adequate information to determine medical necessity as there is no prior functional status listed. Likewise, the statement that the patient requires assistance with clothes management does not indicate if this is a change in status in comparison to his prior status. The pain and swelling in his ankle do not automatically indicate medical necessity. For these clinical findings to be relevant, they must be linked to a functional limitation. For example, if the ankle pain limited his tolerance to weight-

Copyright © Mometrix Media. You have been licensed one copy of this document for personal use only. Any other reproduction or redistribution is strictly prohibited. All rights reserved.
This content is provided for test preparation purposes only and does not imply an endorsement by Mometrix of any particular political, scientific, or religious point of view.

bearing and resulted in a decline in toilet transfer status, it would then be a contributing factor in the determination of medical necessity.

8. C: A person with an avoider sensory pattern functions best with routines and prefers order and consistency. Alone time and small groups are preferred over noisy, crowded activities. A person with a bystander sensory pattern requires extra sensory input to be aware of his or her surroundings. A sensory seeker craves sensory input and prefers new activities over routine activities. A sensor notices everything that is happening in the environment and has difficulty working in a noisy environment.

9. A, D, F: The functional hand position is the safest position when immobilizing the wrist and hand. The functional hand position is 20 degrees of wrist extension with slight ulnar deviation and 60 degrees of metacarpal flexion. Depending on the source, these measurements could vary by 10 degrees.

10. A: A functional job analysis gathers and analyzes data for a specific job versus for a specific person. An occupation-based analysis examines the physical, cognitive, and social demands of a job, taking into consideration the individual's strengths and weaknesses. A risk assessment job analysis is used primarily for injury prevention and health and wellness.

11. C: The stoop lift requires less energy expenditure and less knee flexion range of motion than other types of lifts, such as the traditional lift or deep squat lift. The one-leg stance lift requires good balance and is appropriate only for light lifting of objects that can be easily lifted with one upper extremity. The client may not have adequate balance after bilateral total knee replacements to perform this lift. As a grocery store stocker, his job will require lifting of objects that require use of both upper extremities. The deep squat lift requires a significant amount of knee flexion and would be difficult for this client because of his recent total knee replacements in terms of both range of motion and strength. The half-kneel lift would require weight-bearing through one knee, which would not be tolerated well after a total knee replacement.

12. B: The patient with an acute exacerbation of COPD will present with difficulty breathing and limited endurance related to her diagnosis. Thus, she may not have the endurance to tolerate standing in the shower and require the use of a tub seat. The long-handled sponge would not be necessary for a patient with difficulty breathing. The grab bars would assist with balance; however, in this case scenario, there is no mention of balance issues.

13. A, B, F: Evidence-based practice utilizes up-to-date evidence to guide decisions about the care of individual patients. Interventions should be client centered and actively involve the clients in the intervention process. Evidence-based practice starts with the formulation of a clinical question. Information from personal clinical experience, clinical research, experts, and colleagues all factor into evidence-based practice. Evidence-based practice focuses on client-centered care, not the development of diagnosis-based treatment protocols. Collaborative knowledge is valued. Thus, research from other professions such as psychology, physical therapy, and occupational safety have a place in the evidence-based practice of occupational therapy.

14. D: Systematic reviews summarize the findings of many different research studies that are relevant to the clinical question. The Sackett hierarchy of evidence from most the least supportive is as follows: 1) systematic reviews and meta-analyses of randomized controlled trials; 2) randomized controlled trials; 3) nonrandomized experimental studies; 4) nonexperimental studies; 5) descriptive studies; and 6) respected opinion and expert discussion.

Copyright © Mometrix Media. You have been licensed one copy of this document for personal use only. Any other reproduction or redistribution is strictly prohibited. All rights reserved.
This content is provided for test preparation purposes only and does not imply an endorsement by Mometrix of any particular political, scientific, or religious point of view.

15. B: A patient with a transfemoral amputation is at risk for contractures of the hip flexors and hip abductors. Contractures of the hip flexors and hamstrings are common with transtibial amputations. Contractures of the hip adductors are not typical with either type of amputation.

16. D: Gravitational insecurity is the irrational fear of head movement out of the upright position during challenged balance activities. A common test for gravitational insecurity is to have the child lay supine on a large therapy ball and then to challenge the child's balance by suddenly tipping the ball backward, resulting in sudden head movement. Difficulty stabilizing the shoulders, neck, arms, and trunk as the occupational therapist (OT) attempts to move the child is an indication of decreased proximal stability. Children with abnormal equilibrium or righting reactions will have difficulty sitting on a large therapy ball while the OT tips the ball from side to side. Lifting the head, neck, and trunk against gravity while in the prone position is utilized as a test of trunk extensor strength.

17. C: The bite reflex will diminish at 2 years of age during normal development. The rooting reflex and the suck reflex will diminish at 3–4 months during normal development. The gag reflex does not diminish with age.

18. A: At 12 months of age, the jaw remains stable for tongue and lip movements and for control with chewing. Moving food from side to side in the mouth typically occurs around 24 months of age. At 7–10 months, the development of upper lip downward movement during spoon-feeding occurs.

19. B: The purpose of the group is to provide exposure to food without the pressure of eating the food. Low-stakes activities include art, making snacks, and playing pretend. Answer B would be the least successful activity because it focuses on eating. In this situation, the sharing of foods would introduce textures, smells, and tastes, thus creating a high-stakes situation.

20. B: Patients with macular degeneration lose their central vision, resulting in blank spots in the visual field. Turning the head will assist the patient with macular degeneration to see all the food on the plate. The clock method would be utilized by a patient who is legally blind. Dimming of the lights would be helpful to a patient with cataracts who complains of glare from the lights.

21. A: Cryotherapy is contraindicated in patients with Reynaud's phenomenon because it can cause spasming of the arteries and possibly lead to tissue necrosis. Chronic obstructive pulmonary disease is a respiratory condition and would not be treated by cryotherapy. A patient with a primary diagnosis that is amenable to cryotherapy would not be prevented from cryotherapy treatment if that person has a secondary diagnosis of chronic obstructive pulmonary disease. An acute ankle sprain would be an indication for cryotherapy, not a contraindication. Systemic lupus erythematosus is an autoimmune disorder. At times, cryotherapy may be utilized to control some of the symptoms of systemic lupus erythematosus.

22. C: Serial casting may be effective in the treatment of spasticity in patients with neurological diagnoses such as cerebral palsy, brain injury, or spinal cord injury. Heterotopic ossification should not be treated with aggressive range of motion or serial casting. Due to altered skin integrity, serial casting would not be the best treatment for range of motion limitations due to burns.

23. B, C, D: The patient is allowed to perform activities in the minimal and light MET categories. Washing dishes and putting away groceries fall into the light category. Knitting is categorized as minimal on the MET scale. Preparing a meal, performing upper body cycling, and walking on a treadmill at 2.5 mph are all moderate activities on the MET scale.

Copyright © Mometrix Media. You have been licensed one copy of this document for personal use only. Any other reproduction or redistribution is strictly prohibited. All rights reserved.
This content is provided for test preparation purposes only and does not imply an endorsement by Mometrix of any particular political, scientific, or religious point of view.

24. B, E, F: These symptoms are consistent with autonomic dysreflexia. Autonomic dysreflexia is a medical emergency and requires immediate medical assistance. Exercise should be immediately stopped. Autonomic dysreflexia is accompanied by severe hypertension. Therefore, the patient should be moved to a seated position, if possible, to assist in lowering the blood pressure. Common causes of autonomic dysreflexia include catheter issues, tight clothing, dressing changes, or pain from pressure ulcers. The COTA should try to determine if there is any noxious stimulus, such as an overfull catheter bag or constricting clothing.

25. A: After a burn, a patient will tend to rest the arm in the typical sleeping position with the forearm pronated. Restrictions in the opposite direction (supination) will then develop. Elbow flexion range of motion is more easily maintained than elbow extension range of motion because patients tend to perform daily activities with elbow flexion, such as eating and sleeping. Thus, elbow extension becomes restricted.

26. C: Part C of IDEA deals with early intervention services for infants and toddlers under age 3. Part A provides an introduction to the general provisions and purpose of IDEA. Part B of IDEA deals specifically with children from age 3 to 21. Part D provides general information on topics such as grants, technical assistance, and parent training.

27. B: Medicare Part B is a supplemental insurance that covers medically necessary outpatient services. Medicare Part A covers inpatient care such as acute care, inpatient rehabilitation centers, skilled nursing facilities, as well as home health care. Medicare Part C refers to Medicare Advantage Plans, which are contracted through private insurance companies. Medicare Part D refers to prescription drug coverage.

28. C: Aprosodia relates to an impairment in the ability to perceive the emotional tone of a conversation. It typically occurs with a right hemisphere lesion. Alexia is the inability to comprehend the written word and is most often the result of a left hemisphere lesion. Asymbolia is difficulty in understanding gestures and symbols. It is typically related to a left hemisphere lesion.

29. C: With ideomotor apraxia II, the patient will understand the task and the motor requirements to complete the task, but when she attempts to complete the task, she will complete a similar task instead. Ideational apraxia occurs when the patient does not have the cognitive ability to understand the motor demands of the task. With ideomotor apraxia I, the patient will understand the motor demands of the task but will not be able to recruit the motor plan to actually carry out the task. Dressing apraxia is a type of ideomotor apraxia that specifically relates to the inability to properly perform a dressing task due to impaired body schema perception or impaired perceptual motor skills.

30. B: Rancho Level IV is characterized by agitation and confusion. The patient often behaves inappropriately and has poor attention and poor short-term memory. Rancho Level III is characterized by localized responses in which a patient will respond in a specific manner to a stimulus, but the responses are often delayed and inconsistent. In Rancho Level V, the agitation is lessened in comparison to Level IV, but the confusion and inappropriate responses continue to be noted.

31. D: The most appropriate action would be to bring the concern to the quality improvement committee. The committee would be able to study the situation, including possible causes and possible solutions. It would also be the committee's responsibility to implement and monitor the plan for change. Because the rehab director does not know if the problem stems from late breakfast trays, staffing shortages on the unit, or some other cause, requesting change from the nutrition or

Copyright © Mometrix Media. You have been licensed one copy of this document for personal use only. Any other reproduction or redistribution is strictly prohibited. All rights reserved.
This content is provided for test preparation purposes only and does not imply an endorsement by Mometrix of any particular political, scientific, or religious point of view.

nursing department would not be the first action that should be taken. The chief compliance officer handles complaints that deal with violations of the code of conduct, company policies, and regulatory requirements. There is nothing in this scenario to suggest that any employee is behaving improperly, so the chief compliance officer would not be involved in this situation.

32. A: Transitioning the patient from individual therapy to group therapy would increase the level of cognitive demand by adding a social component to the therapy session whereby the patient is expected to interact with other members of the group. To increase the challenge to the patient, activities should be progressed from more familiar activities to less familiar activities. Cues should be progressed from external cues that are provided by the therapist to internal cues that are provided by oneself.

33. C: This scenario described how the patient executed the solution (the toilet transfer). The scenario did not provide information regarding the different options available (developing possible solutions) or the rationale for choosing to execute the transfer in this particular manner (choosing one best solution). Likewise, the patient did not evaluate the outcome. For example, there is no mention in the scenario as to whether the patient noted any difficulties in the transfer.

34. A, C, D: A patient with a C4 complete spinal cord injury would have full innervation of the upper trapezius, diaphragm, and cervical paraspinal muscles. Paralysis would be noted in the trunk, upper extremities, and lower extremities. Because the patient has head and neck control, he or she would be able to use a head control device and a mouth stick. Due to paralysis of the trunk muscles, he or she would require positional support devices. The patient would not have the necessary upper extremity strength in the shoulders and elbows to use a U-cuff and would not have the necessary upper extremity strength to grasp hand controls. He or she would require a power wheelchair, not a manual wheelchair.

35. B: Picture B is a flexor tendon repair splint. Picture A is a dynamic ulnar nerve splint. Picture C is a dynamic radial palsy splint. Picture D is a functional resting splint.

36. D: For shoulder extension, the supine position would be considered to be the gravity-assisted position. Side lying (with the weak arm on top) would be the gravity-eliminated position. The prone position would be the gravity-resisted position. For a muscle with poor– strength, the muscle is weak and cannot move against gravity, so it would be strengthened in the gravity-eliminated position. In this case, right shoulder extensors would be strengthened in the left side-lying position. The shoulder extensors with fair+ strength are capable of moving against gravity and would be strengthened in the prone position. Therefore, the proper progression would be from left side-lying exercises to prone exercises.

37. C: Due to this client's age and history of diabetes, his surgical wounds may heal slowly and delay prosthetic fitting. Furthermore, his ability to perform physical labor will be comprised, even with bilateral prostheses. For example, he will lack sensory input through prosthetic feet for any activities that require high-level balance such as walking on a construction beam. Given this information, the best assessment for this client would be one that focuses on the potential to do any type of work versus one that focuses on physical job demands and his job description as a construction worker. A vocational evaluation would be most appropriate for this client because it would assess the following factors: physical and psychomotor capacities; intellectual capacities; emotional stability; interests, attitudes, and knowledge of occupational information; aptitudes and achievements; work skill and work tolerances; work habits; work-related capabilities; and job-seeking skills.

Copyright © Mometrix Media. You have been licensed one copy of this document for personal use only. Any other reproduction or redistribution is strictly prohibited. All rights reserved.
This content is provided for test preparation purposes only and does not imply an endorsement by Mometrix of any particular political, scientific, or religious point of view.

38. C: According to the *Occupational Therapy Practice Framework*, a habit is an acquired tendency to automatically respond and perform in certain consistent ways in familiar environments or situations. A routine is a pattern of behavior that is observable, regular, and repetitive and that provides structure for daily life. A routine is embedded in cultural and ecological contexts. A ritual is a symbolic action with spiritual, cultural, or social meaning contributing to the individual's identity. A role is a set of behaviors expected by society and shaped by culture and context that may be further conceptualized and defined by the client.

39. A, C, E: The thumb spica orthosis maintains the thumb in the opposition position and preserves the first web space. The thumb spica orthosis may be utilized in the treatment of median nerve injuries, rheumatoid arthritis, and De Quervain's tendinitis. A resting orthosis is most commonly utilized for patients who have had a cerebrovascular accident. A wrist cock-up orthosis is utilized for radial nerve palsy and carpal tunnel syndrome.

40. C: The rehabilitation approach focuses on abilities versus disabilities. The focus of this approach is to restore a person to a previous state. With regard to occupation, the rehabilitation approach focuses on the occupation and associated performance skills. The biomechanical approach addresses the body structures and associated functions and physical skills. The motor learning approach focuses on the performance of motor functions by utilizing practice and feedback.

41. B: Breath holding commonly occurs during isometric resistive exercises, especially with high-intensity isometric exercises. This breath holding causes a pressor response, leading to a quick increase in blood pressure. Concentric and eccentric exercises are less likely to cause spikes in blood pressure.

42. C: The use of a button board before buttoning a shirt is an example of transfer-of-learning. The neurodevelopmental approach would utilize techniques such as tactile cuing and faciliatory techniques during buttoning activities. The sensory-integration approach would utilize a repetitive movement sequence with the gradual integration of other sensory cues.

43. B: Principle 8 of the OT Code of Conduct states that "certificants shall not electronically post personal health information or anything, including photos, that may reveal a patient's/client's identity or personal or therapeutic relationship." Therefore, even if the client is in the background, he or she may be recognized, which in turn, would reveal a therapeutic relationship. Likewise, HIPAA has similar verbiage to protect the identity of anyone who is receiving health care services. HIPAA requires that health care information be shared only with colleagues who require the information to perform their jobs. If a colleague is not involved in the care of the patient, the video should not be shared.

44. B, D, E: A person who is having an insulin reaction may present with a moist tongue, hunger, and pale skin. Breath would be normal with no odor. Breathing pattern would be normal to shallow. Vomiting would not be present. Fruity breath, labored breathing, and vomiting are more likely to be present with acidosis.

45. B: When a client appears to be in shock, the clinician should place the client in the supine position with the head slightly lower than the legs. To prevent loss of body heat, a light blanket may be placed over the patient, but a heated blanket would not be appropriate in this situation.

46. C: The catheter bag should be placed below the level of the bladder to prevent backflow. The catheter tube should not be stretched as this could dislodge the catheter. Although it is acceptable to empty the catheter bag when it is half-full, it is not necessary to empty it until it is full.

Copyright © Mometrix Media. You have been licensed one copy of this document for personal use only. Any other reproduction or redistribution is strictly prohibited. All rights reserved.
This content is provided for test preparation purposes only and does not imply an endorsement by Mometrix of any particular political, scientific, or religious point of view.

47. A: One of the many benefits of interprofessional collaboration is that it provides professional development and learning opportunities for the professionals. The interprofessional team utilizes a patient-centered rather than a profession-centered approach. Interprofessional collaboration provides an opportunity for members to better understand the skills, expertise, and roles of other professionals, but it does not support cross-training of licensed professionals.

48. A, C, D: Under the supervision of the occupational therapist, a COTA is allowed to perform parts of a screening or parts of the evaluation process. When deemed appropriate by the occupational therapist (OT), the COTA may also supervise an aide for delegated client-related tasks. The selection of appropriate evaluation instruments, interpretation of data, and determination of need for continued occupational therapy services are tasks that the OT performs.

49. C: The medical necessity statement provides information about why the client requires skilled therapy services. This statement is included in the assessment section of the note. The subjective section of the note contains information that the client said. The objective section of the note includes information about the interventions that occurred on that date. The plan section contains information about ongoing therapy, including modifications to the treatment and discharge plans.

50. A: Standardized tests are reliable and valid, producing quantitative results that can be compared to normative data. Modifications to the administrative procedures (changing the way the test is performed) or adaptations to the client population (using a test that was designed for a specific client population with a different population) will affect the results of the test, specifically the validity of the test. The inter-rater reliability of a standardized test is better than the inter-rater reliability of a non-standardized test.

51. D: A supportive environment includes playmates, space, and play objects. In this scenario, the child was interested in play (the motivation for play) and participated in play (play activities) but did not own many toys (lack of supportive environment). Because the child played appropriately with the toys, he or she had the capacity to play.

52. B, C, E: A font size of 12 is appropriate for people with normal vision. For people with low vision, font size should be 14 or greater. Written instructions should be kept simple and at a level that is appropriate for the client's reading comprehension. Clear and relevant pictures are helpful tools, especially for people with low reading levels. Oral instructions allow for conversational dialogue and provide clients with the opportunity to ask questions. Therefore, oral instructions would have a place in this client's health literacy. Teach-back strategies are appropriate tools for determining the client's level of understanding of the educational materials. Due to this client's low vision, written materials should utilize high-contrast print, not low contrast.

53. D: An amputee wheelchair features rear-wheel axles that are positioned two inches posterior to their normal position to widen the base of support and compensate for the loss of lower extremity weight from the amputation. A hemiplegic wheelchair is designed to allow for propulsion of the wheelchair with the unaffected lower extremity. This is accomplished by a seat height two inches lower than the normal seat height. A reclining wheelchair features a seatback that can be reclined to the horizontal position. A sports wheelchair is a low-profile, lightweight wheelchair with a fixed frame. The rear wheels are canted with fixed or adjustable axles.

54. A: Constraint-induced movement therapy is utilized to treat the learned disuse of a body part that occurs with neurological conditions. Out of the four options, cerebral palsy is the only neurological condition. Osteoarthritis is a degenerative orthopedic condition. Rheumatoid arthritis

Copyright © Mometrix Media. You have been licensed one copy of this document for personal use only. Any other reproduction or redistribution is strictly prohibited. All rights reserved.
This content is provided for test preparation purposes only and does not imply an endorsement by Mometrix of any particular political, scientific, or religious point of view.

is an autoimmune condition. Muscular dystrophy is a genetic condition that results in progressive weakness.

55. D: The definition of flows, according to the *Occupational Therapy Practice Framework*, is "uses smooth and fluid arm and wrist movements when interacting with task objects." Moves is defined as "effectively pushes or pulls task objects along a supporting surface, pulls to open or pushes to close doors and drawers, or pushes on wheels to propel a wheelchair." Coordinates is defined as "uses two or more body parts together to manipulate, hold, and/or stabilize task objects without evidence of fumbling task objects and slipping from one's grasp." Lifts is defined as "effectively raises or lifts task objects without evidence of increased effort."

56. C: According to the *Occupational Therapy Practice Framework*, pacing is both a motor skill and a process skill. Initiating and sequencing are both process skills. Coordinating is a motor skill.

57. B: Repetitive gripping activities should be avoided in a patient with trigger finger. Tendon protection techniques, trigger finger splints, and modalities are all appropriate treatments for this diagnosis.

58. A, B, E: Because patients with rheumatoid arthritis are prone to ulnar drift deformities of the hands, they are taught how to modify activities of daily living. These modifications promote radial deviation instead of ulnar deviation. Patients are also taught to avoid positions that put stress on smaller joints and to use the strongest joints and muscles to reduce the stress on the smaller muscles. In this scenario, turning a doorknob to the thumb side would promote radial deviation. Therefore, answer A is correct. However, opening a jar with the left hand would promote ulnar deviation. Therefore, answer F is incorrect. Likewise, answer D is incorrect. To promote radial deviation, the right-handed person should stir in a counterclockwise motion. Normally, a vegetable peeler would be held diagonally across the palm; however, for a patient with rheumatoid arthritis, the peeler should be held parallel to the MCP joints to decrease the stress through the fingers. Therefore, answer C is incorrect. Sliding objects on the kitchen countertop instead of lifting them protects the hands by distributing the workload over several joints. Therefore, answer E is correct. Likewise, lifting with the palms of both hands will also distribute the workload over several joints; therefore, answer B is correct.

59. C: Bilateral upper extremity integration involves the incorporation of the affected arm into an activity to provide the arm with sensory input and to encourage the development of movement sense. Initially the activity is performed by the unaffected arm while the affected arm is receiving the sensory input. As motor function returns to the affected arm, the affected arm begins to take a more active role in the activities, moving from a stabilization role to an assistive role. Constraint-induced movement forces the patient to utilize the affected arm to overcome learned nonuse of the affected upper extremity. Repetitive task practice involves high-intensity repetitions of a task-specific movement. An example would be the performance of repetitive sit-to-stand transfers utilizing both arms to push off of the wheelchair armrests.

60. A: According to the *Occupational Therapy Practice Framework*, a prevention outcome is one that identifies, reduces, or prevents the onset and reduces the incidence of unhealthy conditions, risk factors, diseases, or injuries. In this case, the seating system is preventing further postural deformities. An improvement outcome is designed to promote an increased occupational performance. An enhancement outcome reflects the development of performance skills and performance patterns that augment existing performance in life occupations.

Copyright © Mometrix Media. You have been licensed one copy of this document for personal use only. Any other reproduction or redistribution is strictly prohibited. All rights reserved.
This content is provided for test preparation purposes only and does not imply an endorsement by Mometrix of any particular political, scientific, or religious point of view.

61. A, B, F: Developmentally, this infant has achieved developmental milestones consistent with a 6-month-old. Therefore, the infant is able to voluntarily suck, make babbling sounds, and perform a munching pattern with age-appropriate foods. Commando crawling and independent sitting are milestones associated with late infancy (7–9 months). Inferior pincer grasp is achieved in transitional infancy (10–12 months).

62. B: Picture B demonstrates the inferior pincer grasp. This grasp includes opposition of the thumb and approximation of the thumb to the volar surface of the index finger. This type of grasp develops between 9 and 10 months of age. Picture A demonstrates the palmar grasp, also known as the primitive squeeze grasp. It is characterized by a pronated hand position with flexion of all the fingers to hold an object against the palm. In this type of grasp, the thumb is not utilized. The palmar grasp develops around 5 months of age. Picture C demonstrates the three-jaw chuck grasp. This is an advanced grasp that develops around 1 year of age. In the three-jaw chuck grasp, the wrist is extended and ulnarly deviated. Objects are grasped between two fingers and the thumb.

63. A: A static-tripod pencil grip is acquired around the age of 3 years; therefore, a 6-year-old child with the developmental skills of a 3-year-old would most likely display this type of grip. A dynamic-tripod pencil grip generally develops around 4 years of age. A palmar-supinate grip is developed around 1–2 years of age.

64. C, E, F: Typically, 2-year-old children are able to paste pieces of paper, sort by size, and match basic shapes, such as circles, triangles, and squares. Stacking nine blocks is generally not mastered until 2 ½–3 years of age. Tracing along a thick line and following three-step commands are both skills that are typically mastered between 3 and 3 ½ years of age.

65. B: Patients with osteoporosis are at high risk for vertebral compression fractures. An abrupt onset of thoracic pain after coughing is highly suspicious for a vertebral compression fracture. The COTA should not proceed with any type of treatment due to a significant change in the patient's status. The COTA should notify the occupational therapist of the change in status, so the occupational therapist can determine if the patient requires further medical management before the resumption of occupational therapy services.

66. B: Brunnstrom stage 3 is characterized by associated reactions. An associated reaction is an abnormal increase in muscle tone of the involved extremity that occurs when an activity requires significant effort of the unaffected extremity. Brunnstrom stage 1 is often referred to as the flaccid stage and is characterized by no motion of the affected extremity. Brunnstrom stage 5 is characterized by the ability to voluntarily move the affected extremity out of the synergy pattern. In Brunnstrom stage 7, the patient is able to perform individual finger movements on the affected extremity.

67. A: Computer workstation ergonomics involve the maintenance of optimal seated posture. The optimal seated posture consists of hips flexed to 90–110 degrees, downward eye gaze of 17–18 degrees, elbows flexed to 90–100 degrees, and wrists in neutral position or less than 30 degrees of flexion or extension.

68. C: The standing time involved in preparing a full meal would be more than the time required to wash the breakfast dishes. Therefore, this task progression is an example of grading of endurance. Advancing from buttoning large buttons to small buttons would be an example of grading of coordination. Because a bag of flour weighs more than a plate, advancing from lifting a plate to lifting a bag of flour would be an example of grading of strength.

Copyright © Mometrix Media. You have been licensed one copy of this document for personal use only. Any other reproduction or redistribution is strictly prohibited. All rights reserved.
This content is provided for test preparation purposes only and does not imply an endorsement by Mometrix of any particular political, scientific, or religious point of view.

69. B: Poor splint design and fit can lead to pressure areas. Proximal and distal edges of the splint should be flared to reduce pressure areas. The splint size should be two-thirds the length of the forearm. Internal and external corners should be rounded. Angular corners are sharp and may dig into the patient's skin.

70. B: At 3 years of age, a child should be able to hold up the correct number of fingers to identify his or her age. Manipulating a squeeze bottle generally occurs around 4 ½–5 years of age. Using table utensils skillfully usually occurs around 4–4 ½ years of age.

71. C: Occupational Safety and Health Administration (OSHA) annual training is a requirement of the facility that is mandatory for the facility's accreditation status. The annual training is not considered to be an acceptable form of professional development in terms of continuing competency. Likewise, corporate compliance training is not considered to be an acceptable form of professional development in terms of continuing competency. CPR training and certification are considered to be an acceptable competency for license renewal.

72. B, C, D: A stage one pressure wound is defined as erythema that does not blanch when pressure is applied. A stage one wound is not an open wound. The treatment of a stage one wound focuses on prevention. Treatment should relieve pressure through mechanisms such as pressure-relieving cushions and positioning schedules. Treatment also focuses on prevention of infection by keeping the area clean. Avoidance of shearing forces prevents progression of the wound to stage two. Absorption of exudate is involved in the treatment of an infected wound or a draining wound. Removal of eschar is involved in the treatment of necrotic tissue in stage four or five wounds. Maintenance of a moist wound bed is appropriate for open wounds, such as stage two to four wounds.

73. B: For a posterolateral approach to a total hip replacement, the patient should avoid crossing the surgical leg across midline (adduction) and avoid internal rotation. The ideal position of the affected hip in the supine position would be slight abduction and neutral rotation.

74. A: The Clinical Test for Sensory Interaction in Balance (CTSIB) has six different sensory test conditions. The first condition is normal standing with eyes open and a stable surface, which is used as the baseline. The next five conditions systematically vary sensory inputs, resulting in sensory conflict and postural difficulty. The condition that maximally challenges a patient with vestibular dysfunction would be condition #6, which is the most difficult condition. In condition #6, visual conflict occurs with moving surroundings and a moving platform.

75. C: Figure-ground discrimination is the ability to visually distinguish a figure from the background. During laundry tasks, a person with impaired figure-ground discrimination would have difficulty finding socks amidst other laundry. Form discrimination is the ability to group and to differential forms of the same item and to identify an item when it is viewed from a different angle or perspective. Depth perception is the ability to recognize and understand differences in distances between objects.

76. B: Universal design is "the design of environments and products to be usable by all people to the greatest extent possible without the need for special arrangements or adaptations; intended to simplify life for everyone by making products, communications, and the built environment more usable by as many people as possible or little or no extra cost." Equitable use is a principle of universal design. Universal design does not utilize the cost-saving measure of using low-end building supplies. Because universal design focuses on creating a design that can be used by as many people as possible, customization of size and space is not a principle of universal design.

Copyright © Mometrix Media. You have been licensed one copy of this document for personal use only. Any other reproduction or redistribution is strictly prohibited. All rights reserved.
This content is provided for test preparation purposes only and does not imply an endorsement by Mometrix of any particular political, scientific, or religious point of view.

77. C: When ambulating with a patient, the clinician should stand in a posterolateral position in relationship to the patient with one hand on the gait belt. The opposite hand may be placed on the patient's shoulder but should not be placed on the upper extremity as this hand position has the potential to cause injury to a patient during a fall. The clinician should move in step with the patient, maintaining a wide base of support, which improves stability.

78. D: Sink height should be 32–34 inches from the floor. Ramps should have a maximum of 1:12 ramp slope ratio. Door width should be 32 inches at minimum, preferably 36 inches. Bed height should be 18–22 inches from the floor.

79. A: Sensory processing disorder (SPD) is a disorder that is characterized by difficulty receiving, processing, and appropriately responding to sensory information from the environment and the body. All of the answer choices are appropriate interventions for SPD; however, play-based vestibular activities would be a direct treatment intervention, not a lifestyle accommodation. Changing the lighting source would be an example of an environmental modification, not a lifestyle accommodation. Providing the child with seamless clothes with the tags removed would be an example of a lifestyle accommodation.

80. B, C, F: Redirection of an adult in a group setting should be as subtle and inconspicuous as possible. Using proximity will sometimes settle down a disruptive person. Drawing the person into the group activity by asking a question or giving responsibility can help engage the person. Because the goal of the redirection is to avoid further disruption to the group, the redirection should not be used as a teaching moment for the group, to distract the group by use of an authoritative tone of voice, or to enlist the help of other participants.

81. D: A Bankart lesion is an injury to the anterior glenoid labrum and is associated with an anterior shoulder dislocation. An anterior shoulder dislocation is most likely to occur in a position that includes shoulder external rotation and abduction to 90 degrees. This position overloads the anterior capsule and allows the humeral head to translate forward.

82. C: The picture demonstrates strengthening of the external rotator muscles of the shoulder. Although all of the answer choices are muscles of the rotator cuff, the teres minor is a key external rotator. The supraspinatus muscle is most active is during the initiation of shoulder abduction. The subscapularis muscle functions as an internal rotator of the shoulder.

83. A: The optimal position for a tendon during friction massage is in the lengthened position. Friction massage is performed perpendicular to the tendon.

84. D: Patients are taught to dress in a manner that conserves energy while promoting safety. The lower body should be dressed first. Socks should be donned before pants to assure that the socks will fit under the pant legs. After the socks are donned, the next step is to put on undergarments, followed by pants, then shoes. Once the lower body is dressed, the shirt is donned.

85. B: A patient weighing more than 300 pounds will require a bariatric wheelchair. Due to pain and range of motion restrictions associated with the recent total knee replacement, the wheelchair should have elevating leg rests. For safety, the bariatric patient requires a two-person assist level.

86. D: A mechanical lift such as a Hoyer lift is the best option because it is appropriate for dependent patients and can be used to transfer a patient safely from a bed to a wheelchair. An air-assistive device is appropriate for lateral, dependent transfers from a supine position on a bed to a supine position on a gurney but not to a wheelchair. A sliding board and a stand-lift device are both

Copyright © Mometrix Media. You have been licensed one copy of this document for personal use only. Any other reproduction or redistribution is strictly prohibited. All rights reserved.
This content is provided for test preparation purposes only and does not imply an endorsement by Mometrix of any particular political, scientific, or religious point of view.

appropriate transfer devices but are used with patients who are able to partially assist with the transfer.

87. A: A patient with a spinal cord injury at the C7 level will have triceps strength and be able to partially assist with transfers. The patient with the C5 level injury will require more assistance. According to the ASIA scale, grade A is a complete spinal cord injury with a lack of motor and sensory function below the level of injury. Grade E on the ASIA scale indicates a return to normal strength in a previously impaired segment. Therefore, the patient with the most significant impairment would be the patient with the C5 ASIA A spinal cord injury (answer A).

88. C: Postoperative rotator cuff protocols, devised by surgeons, are utilized to determine progression of exercise. In the early phases of rehabilitation, passive range of motion is performed in the scapular plane to avoid impingement. External rotation and elevation in the scapular plane are the first two motions to be regained. The CPM machine would be utilized for these two motions. By the time the patient can progress to other motions, the CPM would no longer be indicated.

89. B, D, F: Of the choices listed, the best rationales for clinical documentation are continuity of care among rehab professionals, chronological record of care, and reimbursement requirements. Continuity of care is a broad term that encompasses any clinical activity related to the patient's care on both a short-term and a long-term basis. Continuity of care dictates that the patient receives high quality of care over the course of time. Examples of continuity of care could include supervision of the COTA by the occupational therapist, transitional care from one type of rehabilitation setting to another, and coverage of the patient's treatment session by a different clinician, such as for vacation leave. As a chronological record of care, clinical documentation provides a record of the patient's status with regard to medical diagnoses, treatments, response to treatment, progress, and future needs. This chronological record of care is vital in the ongoing care of the patient over time. Last, clinical documentation is also utilized to determine skilled level of care and other insurance requirements related to reimbursement. Community resources are adjuncts to medical treatment that are provided by programs within the community. Examples may include Meals on Wheels, support groups, transportation services, or financial assistance. Although certain relevant information about a patient may be provided to the community resource with the patient's permission, the clinical documentation in its entirety is not provided. Although an exercise log is part of the occupational therapy documentation, it is not a rationale for clinical documentation but, rather, a component of the chronological record of care. At times, patients may request access to their clinical information or gain access to certain documents through a patient portal system. However, the patient is not a key target audience for clinical documentation that utilizes complex medical terminology. More often than not, patients are provided with overview summaries that are written in patient-friendly terminology. Examples include visit summaries, discharge instructions, and follow-up instructions. In the event that the patient is seeking access to large portions of clinical documentation for legal reasons, this would then fall under the rationale of clinical documentation as a legal record.

90. A: According to the Individuals with Disabilities Education Act (IDEA), goals should be developed by a team approach. Goals should be student centered and focus on a functional outcome within the educational setting that is addressed by several members of the team versus occupational therapy (OT)-specific goals. Goals should be worded to indicate what the student will do and under what conditions the skill will be performed. Answer choice A is the best answer that fits this description. In answer choices B and D, the wording is not student centered but, rather, focuses on what the OT staff will do. Answer choice C indicates that improvement will be determined by a score on a standardized test. Although this would be a reliable indicator of

Copyright © Mometrix Media. You have been licensed one copy of this document for personal use only. Any other reproduction or redistribution is strictly prohibited. All rights reserved.
This content is provided for test preparation purposes only and does not imply an endorsement by Mometrix of any particular political, scientific, or religious point of view.

functional improvement, it does not provide a specific functional activity that would be noted within the educational setting.

91. B, C, E: The typical upper extremity flexor pattern consists of scapular depression and retraction, shoulder adduction and internal rotation, elbow flexion, wrist flexion and ulnar deviation, and finger flexion. When the elbow presents with increased flexor tone of the biceps muscle, the clinician would want to facilitate the triceps, the antagonist muscle, through tactile stimulation. When the affected hand is essentially held in a fisted position due to increased flexor tone of the fingers, the clinician would attempt to relax the tone by passively moving the fingers into relative extension. To do this, the clinician would grasp either the pinky finger or the thumb to open the hand. When the hand is fisted, the clinician would not be able to move the three middle fingers, digits 2, 3, and 4. Another technique to open a fisted hand is for the clinician to put his or her hand into the patient's hand. Because the pattern of tone at the wrist is into flexion and ulnar deviation, the clinician would introduce his or her hand to the ulnar aspect of the patient's hand to break up the ulnar hypertonicity.

92. B: Parallel participation occurs when group members work side by side in a supportive manner, but there is little to no interaction among group members, although the members are aware of each other. Associative participation occurs when group members exchange brief interactions such as greeting one another or making small talk. Cooperation and competition begin to be demonstrated by the group members. Members are focused on the task but start to give and receive minimal assistance to and from other group members. Supportive cooperative participation emphasizes camaraderie and emotional sharing around a task. The task is considered secondary to the emotional support. Members demonstrate growth in personal and interpersonal insight. Mature participation occurs when members take turns in acting as teacher, learner, and mentor. Members balance the social-emotional needs of the group members with the completion of the task.

93. C: Neurodevelopmental Treatment (NDT) utilizes physical handling techniques and key points of control to support body segments and assist the patient in regaining active control. Answer choice A describes the Rood approach, whereas answer choice B describes proprioceptive neuromuscular facilitation (PNF).

94. B: A patient with rheumatoid arthritis will have difficulty with prolonged gripping activities. Therefore, the most beneficial card-playing adaptation would be the card holder. The patient with rheumatoid arthritis might have decreased coordination due to rheumatoid deformities and benefit from the card sorter; however, this item would not be as necessary as the card holder. Also, in a group setting, someone else would be available to shuffle the cards. The large-size cards would not be helpful to this patient because the diameter of the cards is the issue, not the overall size. The large size cards would be most appropriate for someone with low vision.

95. A, C, D: The radial styloid process, the ulnar styloid process, and the thumb web space are the areas that are most likely to develop pressure points when wearing a wrist immobilizer splint. The lateral epicondyle is located at the elbow. The splint will not extend far enough proximally to cause pressure at the elbow. Likewise, the wrist immobilization splint should not extend far enough distally to cause pressure to either the metacarpal or proximal phalange of the thumb.

96. A: A contrast bath is the most appropriate choice of a modality to address subacute edema of the whole hand. The contrast bath involves alternating between dipping the hand in warm water and in cold water, thereby alternating vasodilation and vasoconstriction. Because this modality utilizes water, all areas of the hand will be in contact with the modality. Cold packs are appropriate for the treatment of edema, especially acute edema; however, this is not the ideal modality for this

Copyright © Mometrix Media. You have been licensed one copy of this document for personal use only. Any other reproduction or redistribution is strictly prohibited. All rights reserved.
This content is provided for test preparation purposes only and does not imply an endorsement by Mometrix of any particular political, scientific, or religious point of view.

case scenario because it would be difficult to maintain contact between the cold pack and all the contours of the hand. The transcutaneous electrical nerve stimulation (TENS) unit is most appropriate in the treatment of pain and has not been validated as an appropriate modality for subacute edema.

97. C: Thrombophlebitis is a contraindication to the use of heat because the increased tissue temperature could cause a blood clot to become dislodged and travel to a vital organ, potentially leading to death. Pregnancy is a precaution for the use of heat. Although full body heating, such as a warm whirlpool, is not recommended during pregnancy, a hot pack to the knee of a pregnant woman is an acceptable treatment. Cardiac insufficiency is a precaution to the use of heat because heat can cause local and generalized vasodilation, which can contribute to increased cardiac demand. However, heat can be used with caution for a cardiac patient but discontinued if the patient feels faint or experiences a decrease in blood pressure.

98. B: Neuromuscular electrical stimulation is effective in increasing muscle strength in orthopedic conditions as well as improving motor control in patients with central nervous system conditions such as a stroke. Direct current electrical muscle stimulation is used in the treatment of denervated muscle due to nerve injury or disease. Transcutaneous electrical nerve stimulation is used to modulate pain.

99. D: Compression, such as customized compression garments, elastic bandages, wraps, or tubular elastic cotton supports, is the best treatment for hypertrophic scarring. Positioning, stretching, and massage are all appropriate adjunctive treatments to use in addition to compression.

100. C: A large dispersive pad of opposite polarity should be placed on intact skin several inches away from the wound. The dispersive pad does not actively treat the wound; it completes the electrical circuit.

101. C: Encouraging the child to suck on an ice pop is one technique to promote swallowing in children. Toddlers and adolescents should be positioned in the upright sitting position with the neck slightly flexed. Only infants should feed in the semi-reclined position. Verbal cues can be distracting and should be avoided as much as possible.

102. B: Relational play occurs when an infant understands the function of an object then uses the object accordingly. Stacking blocks is an example of relational play. Banging a rattle is an example of sensorimotor play. In this early form of play, infants perform activities because they enjoy the physical sensation that is created. Making a pretend meal is an example of symbolic play.

103. D: A plate switch can be activated with a light touch and is the most appropriate option for a child with minimal hand movement and poor strength. A button switch requires the child to press down on the switch then release it. A grasp switch requires the child to squeeze and release the switch. A ribbon switch requires the child to be able to reach and swipe with fair accuracy to engage it.

104. A: An injury to the ulnar nerve will result in weakness of the intrinsic muscles, leading to a claw position of the ring and small finger. The anti-claw splint is the best splint option for this type of injury.

105. C: Attention refers to sustained attention and concentration. Meal preparation requires a significant amount of attention to safety. A lack of attention could result in burning food or a fire. Thought function refers to the control and content of thought such as the awareness of reality. Experience of self and time refers to one's emotional status related to body image and self-concept.

Copyright © Mometrix Media. You have been licensed one copy of this document for personal use only. Any other reproduction or redistribution is strictly prohibited. All rights reserved.
This content is provided for test preparation purposes only and does not imply an endorsement by Mometrix of any particular political, scientific, or religious point of view.

Emotional functions refer to the regulation and appropriateness of emotions. Thought, emotion, and experience of self and time functions are not relevant to this particular task.

106. A: Donning socks and shoes typically involves crossing the lower extremity beyond midline and/or bending more than 90 degrees at the hip, which would break hip precautions. Donning a bra and shirt can be completed safely by a patient on hip precautions. Brushing teeth and washing dishes both involve prolonged standing and slight bending at the trunk. Although these activities may be uncomfortable or difficult for a patient with a recent hip replacement, they can be completed safely by a patient on hip precautions.

107. B: Consultation involves the use of one's knowledge and skills as an expert in a given field to provide others with information to guide decision-making. In this case, the occupational therapist and COTA are serving as consultants to the school administration team. A training approach provides information and practice opportunities to enhance a skill or process. An advocate would use persuasion to change the opinion of other people. A prevention approach would focus on strategies to prevent injury, disease, or disability.

108. A: The safe position is commonly used during splint fabrication after burns, trauma, and invasive surgery. The safe position maintains optimal stress on the metacarpal, phalangeal, and IP collateral ligaments. The safe position consists of MP joints in flexion, IP joints in full extension, and the wrist in 10–30 degrees of extension. The resting position is the position that the hand normally maintains at rest and consists of 10–20 degrees of wrist extension, all finger joints in slight flexion, and the thumb positioned midway between opposition and abduction with the pad facing the side of the index finger. The resting position maintains the proximal, distal, and longitudinal arches and is often used in resting splints or splints that prevent deformity. The functional position of the hand is the position of the hand that occurs with most activity and consists of 20–30 degrees of wrist extension, thumb abduction and opposition to the pad of the middle finger, 30 degrees of metacarpal flexion, and 45 degrees of IP joint flexion. In the functional position, tension is equal in all muscles, and the hand is mechanically efficient.

109. C: Choreiform movements are uncontrolled, irregular, purposeless, quick, jerky, dysrhythmic movements. Athetoid movements are slow, wormlike, arrhythmic movements, usually occurring in the distal extremities. Ballistic movements are also known as projectile movements and are characterized by continuous, gross, abrupt contractions of the axial and proximal muscles of the extremity.

110. B, C, F: The neutral position is the position in which the body functions most efficiently. In standing, the neutral position consists of shoulders positioned at one's sides, elbows flexed to 90 degrees, forearms in neutral position, wrists straight, back straight with maintenance of normal curves, hips extended, and knees slightly flexed.

111. B: When a person is having a seizure, the immediate area should be cleared of objects that could cause injury. The person should not be held down. It is appropriate to attempt to keep the person's airway open, but objects should not be placed in the mouth.

112. A: Desensitization techniques include the use of textures for tactile input. To provide adequate input, textures are progressed from soft textures, such as cotton balls, to rough textures, such as wool or a paper towel. Submersion of the hand in a container of rice or other textured items would be appropriate, but warm water will not have a significant effect on hypersensitivity. Passive range of motion techniques are appropriate to regain motion in the affected finger but are not a component of the desensitization intervention.

Copyright © Mometrix Media. You have been licensed one copy of this document for personal use only. Any other reproduction or redistribution is strictly prohibited. All rights reserved.
This content is provided for test preparation purposes only and does not imply an endorsement by Mometrix of any particular political, scientific, or religious point of view.

113. C: The specific location of the nerve injury will determine which muscles are affected. Injury to the median nerve at the level of the wrist would result in the inability to flex the thumb tip and index fingertip to the palm of the hand. Injury to the radial nerve could result in weakness or paralysis of the triceps, brachioradialis, supinator, extensor carpi radialis longus, and/or extensor carpi radialis brevis, depending on the location of the injury. An ulnar nerve injury could affect the flexor carpi ulnaris, the median half of the flexor digitorum profundus, and the intrinsic muscles of the hand.

114. B: A boxer's fracture is a fracture of the fourth or fifth metacarpal. A Bennett fracture is a fracture of the palmar base of the proximal first metacarpal. A Colles' fracture is a fracture of the distal end of the radius. A Smith fracture is also known as a reverse Colles' fracture and occurs to the distal radius during a fall on the dorsum of the hand.

115. C: A mallet finger is the result of damage to the extensor mechanism, resulting in a flexed position of the distal interphalangeal (DIP) joint. A Boutonniére deformity is caused by damage to the central tendon and triangular ligament at the proximal interphalangeal (PIP) joint. The resultant deformity involves flexion position at the PIP joint and hyperextension of the DIP joint. Dupuytren contracture is a flexion contracture of the metacarpal phalangeal (MCP) joint. Most commonly the fourth and/or fifth digits are involved.

116. C: Handling characteristics are the characteristics of the splint material that allow the material to be handled during the forming process. Performance characteristics are the characteristics of the material that relate to the use of the splint once it has hardened. Of the three answer choices, only Answer C (elasticity) relates to the handling of the material during the forming process. Rigidity and durability are performance characteristics.

117. A: Ultrasound is appropriate in the treatment of subacute inflammation. Edema is treated with cryotherapy, which promotes vasoconstriction. Spasticity is a tightness in muscles that results from a central nervous system problem. Ultrasound is not the treatment of choice for spasticity.

118. D: An avulsion fracture is caused by a traction force exerted by a ligament or tendon in which a small part of the bone is pulled off. A stress fracture is a small crack in a bone that is caused by repetitive microtrauma. A Greenstick fracture is a type of fracture that occurs in children due to a bending of the bone. A pathological fracture is a fracture that occurs due to a disease state such as cancer or osteoporosis.

119. C, E, F: Performance of active ankle pumping exercises, use of a sequential pneumatic compression unit while in bed, and wearing of compression stockings are all appropriate interventions to prevent the development of a deep vein thrombosis. Early ambulation is encouraged after surgery. Prolonged sitting should be avoided. Legs should be elevated in sitting or supine.

120. C: The Individuals with Disabilities Education Improvement Act (IDEA) states that children with disabilities should receive their education in the least restrictive environment. IDEA defines the least restrictive environment as "the environment that provides maximum interaction with nondisabled peers and is consistent with the needs of the child/student."

121. B: An engineering control is a change to the equipment or physical demands of a job. Use of a pneumatic lifting device fits into this category. Ear plugs would be an example of personal protective equipment (PPE) controls. Mandatory work breaks are an example of administrative and work practice controls.

Copyright © Mometrix Media. You have been licensed one copy of this document for personal use only. Any other reproduction or redistribution is strictly prohibited. All rights reserved.
This content is provided for test preparation purposes only and does not imply an endorsement by Mometrix of any particular political, scientific, or religious point of view.

122. A: A metal, double-upright AFO inserts into the sides of the sole of the shoe. The only direct point of contact with the skin is the strap that is located distal to the fibular head. Both the prefabricated and custom plastic AFOs are designed as total-contact AFOs and do not accommodate fluctuations in edema well. The type of ankle, solid versus hinged, is determined by the amount of stability and assistance that is required at the ankle.

123. A,B,E: Areas of occupation include activities of daily living, instrumental activities of daily living, rest and sleep, education, work, play, leisure, and social participation. Habits, routines, and rituals are examples of performance patterns.

124. D: The scaphoid lies within the anatomical snuffbox.

125. B, D, E: Treatment of a wound may utilize electrical stimulation, whirlpool, or ultrasound. The technique for the treatment of a wound will be modified for electrical stimulation and ultrasound to avoid contamination of the wound. Open wounds should not be submersed in a paraffin bath or into a fluidotherapy machine. Cold packs are used to treat pain, edema, and spasticity but are not appropriate for the treatment of open wounds.

126. B, C, F: Instrumental activities of daily living (IADLs) are activities involving the environment. They are considered to be optional activities, meaning that it is possible to not be required to perform these activities in one's life. For example, money management is an IADL. In many households, only one person may be responsible for the management of the finances. Of the activities listed, community mobility, financial management, and meal preparation are IADLs. On the other hand, activities of daily living (ADLs) are activities that involve taking care of one's own body and self. Functional mobility (movements required to take care of oneself), toileting, and eating are examples of ADLs.

127. B: Material safety data sheets (MSDS) are written instructions from the chemical's manufacturer that outlines procedures to follow when using the chemical, including the use of personal protective equipment. The Occupational Safety and Health Administration (OSHA) requires all toxic chemicals and flammable substances to have an MSDS. Universal precautions are a set of guidelines designed to prevent transmission of pathogens to others. Examples of infection control policies include disinfection and sterilization, environmental infection control, hand hygiene, and isolation precautions.

128. C: The ability to swallow, open the mouth, and close the mouth are examples of movement functions. Sequencing the movement of the brush is an example of a cognitive function. Feeling of the water and brush in the mouth is an example of a sensory function.

129. B: The levator scapula muscle is innervated by the dorsal scapular nerve. The trapezius muscle is innervated by the 11th cranial nerve, known as the spinal accessory nerve. The serratus anterior muscle is innervated by the long thoracic nerve. The pectoralis minor muscle is innervated by the median pectoral nerve.

130. D, E, F: The *Occupational Therapy Practice Framework* breaks down the category of body functions into eight broad categories. The mental functions category is one of these broad categories. Within the mental functions' category are eight subcategories: higher-level cognition, attention, memory, perception, thought, sequencing complex movement, emotional, and experience of self and time. Judgement, praxis, and insight are all types of higher-level cognitive functions. Visual discrimination is an example of a perception function. Logical thought is a thought function. Concentration belongs in the attention function category.

Copyright © Mometrix Media. You have been licensed one copy of this document for personal use only. Any other reproduction or redistribution is strictly prohibited. All rights reserved.
This content is provided for test preparation purposes only and does not imply an endorsement by Mometrix of any particular political, scientific, or religious point of view.

131. A: The *Occupational Therapy Practice Framework* outlines nine types of outcomes: occupational performance, adaptation, health and wellness, participation, prevention, quality of life, role competence, self-advocacy, and occupational justice. Participation involves the engagement in occupations that are meaningful, personally fulfilling, and harmonious with cultural expectations. Attendance at a church service is an example of a participation outcome. Prevention is the creation of conditions for a healthy lifestyle and health promotion. This outcome does not fit well with the activity of attending church. Quality of life involves a client's sense of hope, satisfaction, perception of self, and health and well-being. This outcome is somewhat ambiguous and difficult to measure. In the scenario of attending church, there is not enough information about the client's socio-emotional status to justify this type of outcome. Adaptation is the ability to find an alternative way to do something. This outcome does not correlate well with the described scenario.

132. D: Camptodactyly is a congenital medical condition that involves a flexion deformity of the proximal interphalangeal joints of the hand. Although other fingers may be involved, the little finger is always involved.

133. A, D, F: A standardized test is a test that is administered and scored in a consistent manner. A norm-referenced test is a subcategory of the standardized test. In a norm-referenced test, the test is first given to a large number of individuals by the creator of the test to serve as a normative sample. Therapists then can give the test to their patients and compare the patients' performance to the normative data on subjects of similar qualities such as age. Criterion-referenced tests are another subcategory of standardized test. In a criterion-referenced test, a list of criteria is developed by the creator of the test. This list of criteria is based on a standard sample of the population and is used to evaluate patients against the criteria. The following characteristics are true of the norm-based test: requires diagnostic skills, maximizes differences among individuals, and evaluates individual performance against a group. These characteristics are true of a criterion-referenced test: depends on task analysis, utilizes cutoff scores, and is sensitive to the effects of therapy.

134. A: The Functional Independence Measure (FIM) is a criterion-referenced, 18-item test that provides a uniform system of measurement for disability. It is commonly used in the inpatient rehabilitation setting. The Canadian Occupational Performance Measure (COPM) utilizes a semi-structured interview process to obtain the clients' perception of self-care status, productivity, social participation, and leisure. The Melville-Nelson Self-Care Assessment (SCA) is commonly used in the subacute rehabilitation setting and the skilled nursing home setting. The SCA provides a means to objectively analyze a patient's self-care status within the scope of Medicare guidelines.

135. C: Prevention programs can be classified as primary, secondary, or tertiary. The classification is based on the timing of the intervention relative to the health condition. A primary prevention is one that prevents people from getting a disease or injury. Vaccines are an example of primary prevention. Secondary prevention describes interventions that minimize the duration, severity, and sequelae of a health condition. Health screenings such as colonoscopies, mammograms, and blood pressure monitoring are examples of secondary prevention. Tertiary prevention occurs after the health condition has been diagnosed and is geared toward adaptation, accommodation, and rehabilitation. An aquatic exercise program would be an example of a tertiary prevention program.

136. B: Due to the recent surgery on the right leg, the patient is at risk for the development of a deep vein thrombosis (DVT). The signs and symptoms in the scenario are consistent with a DVT. A DVT is considered to be a medical emergency due to the possibility that it could embolize to vital organs, such as the lungs, resulting in death if it is not treated. The appropriate action for the COTA would be to stop treatment and notify the evaluating occupational therapist (OT). It is appropriate for the OT to contact the doctor immediately, but it is not appropriate for the patient to notify the

Copyright © Mometrix Media. You have been licensed one copy of this document for personal use only. Any other reproduction or redistribution is strictly prohibited. All rights reserved.
This content is provided for test preparation purposes only and does not imply an endorsement by Mometrix of any particular political, scientific, or religious point of view.

doctor on the following day. Modification to treatment is not the most appropriate option because this is a life-threatening condition.

137. B: Level II of the dysphagia diet consists of mechanically altered foods. Finely chopped meat would be an example of a mechanically altered food. Level I foods are pureed. Level III foods include foods that are naturally soft and near regular texture. Hard, dry, sticky, or crunchy foods are not allowed. Level IV is a regular diet and includes all foods.

138. C, D, F: Exercises for the oral stage of swallowing include tongue range of motion, jaw range of motion, and lip-resistive exercises. Tongue base retraction exercises, shaker exercises, and pitch exercises are examples of exercises to promote the pharyngeal stage of swallowing.

139. D: A self-perception scale utilizes a questionnaire that is completed by the patient and provides insight into the patient's deficits through the patient's report of past experiences and associated perceptions. The Falls Efficacy Scale utilizes a 1–10 scale. The patients rate their confidence in their ability to perform a list of activities without falling. None of the other answer choices utilize a self-perception scale.

140. A, B, C: In the mental health setting, the interdisciplinary team generally consists of the following health care professionals: psychiatrist, registered and licensed practical nurse, nurse aide, social worker, and occupational therapy practitioner. Psychiatrists generally are the team leaders in the mental health setting and are responsible for admitting and discharging clients, prescribing and monitoring medication use, and providing individual and group psychotherapy. The social worker is responsible for assessing family dynamics and providing community resource information to the client and/or family. The occupational therapy practitioner leads group activities and assesses clients' functional status and skills through daily structured activities. Generally, physical therapy and speech therapy services are not provided in the mental health setting unless a comorbidity exists that would necessitate their services. Last, although the emergency room physician may be the first point of contact for a client, such as the case with attempted suicide, the emergency room doctor's involvement ends as soon as the client leaves the emergency room setting.

141. A: Coban should be applied from distal to proximal to promote lymph flow. Active exercise is allowed while wearing a Coban wrap. The wrap should be snug but should not be pulled as tight as possible because this can impede circulation.

142. B: The mechanical elbow of a transhumeral prosthesis is controlled by tension in the cable. To create tension in the cable and flex the mechanical elbow, the scapula is abducted, and the shoulder is flexed.

143. C: Back pain is a common age-related skeletal problem for adults. Scoliosis is a concern during rapid times of growth that occurs during adolescence. Osteoporosis and osteoarthritis are conditions that are associated with older adulthood. During older adulthood, peak bone mass decreases, leading to osteoporosis. Osteoarthritis is an age-related condition due to the degeneration of articular cartilage in joints. This degeneration occurs over time, leading to pain and physical limitations during older adulthood.

144. A: Astereognosis is a perceptual deficit in which the person is unable to identify familiar objects through touch, proprioception, and cognition without the use of vision. In this scenario, the patient's vision is obscured by the soap suds and he or she must rely on tactile input to identify the objects. Visual agnosia is an inability to accurately identify everyday objects that are seen. The person with visual agnosia can see the object but cannot accurately name the object. Apraxia is the

Copyright © Mometrix Media. You have been licensed one copy of this document for personal use only. Any other reproduction or redistribution is strictly prohibited. All rights reserved.
This content is provided for test preparation purposes only and does not imply an endorsement by Mometrix of any particular political, scientific, or religious point of view.

inability to plan and perform motor acts even though adequate motor control and strength are present.

145. B: Balance is maintained by keeping the center of gravity over the base of support. There are three main strategies used by adults to recover balance in response to sudden perturbations. These strategies are the ankle strategy, the hip strategy, and the stepping strategy. For small perturbations, movements at the ankle, known as ankle strategies, are sufficient to bring the center of gravity back over the base of support. For quick or large perturbations, the hip strategy is needed to realign the center of gravity over the base of support. When a large force displaces the center of gravity beyond the limits of stability, a stepping strategy is required to realign the center of gravity over the base of support.

146. A, B, D: After a total shoulder arthroplasty, the following activities must be avoided in the first 4–6 weeks: combined shoulder extension and internal rotation, such as reaching behind the back; lifting more than 1 pound; and weight-bearing through the involved arm, such as pushing up from a chair. Light isometric exercise of the deltoid and scapulothoracic muscles, passive range of motion up to 30 degrees of external rotation, and writing with the elbow at waist level are allowed during the first 4–6 weeks after surgery.

147. B: A swan-neck deformity consists of hyperextension of the PIP joints and flexion of the DIP joints. After surgical correction, a static splint would prevent these positions. Therefore, splinting would incorporate flexion at the PIP joints and extension of the DIP joints. Of all the answer choices, only Answer B includes flexion of the PIP joints and extension of the DIP joints.

148. C: In this case scenario, the patient needs to build muscular endurance. Exercise performance with low resistance and increasing the number of repetitions or the amount of time are methods for grading exercises to improve muscular endurance. Exercise performance with increasing levels of resistance and low repetitions is a method for grading exercises to improve muscle strength. Exercise performance with increasing amounts of resistance while shortening the time period is a method for grading exercises to improve muscle power.

149. A: Relative increases in blood pressure and heart rate are normal responses to exercise. Exercise should be discontinued if systolic blood pressure reaches 200 mm Hg. A 15 mm Hg increase in systolic blood pressure is acceptable with exercise. Exercise should be discontinued if diastolic blood pressure reaches 110 mm Hg. With exercise, diastolic blood pressure usually stays the same, increases up to 10 mm Hg, or decreases up to 10 mm Hg. A 20 beats/minute increase in heart rate from resting heart rate is normal. Any drop of heart rate with exercise is considered an inappropriate response to exercise.

150. B: The lumbrical muscles flex the metacarpophalangeal joints and extend the interphalangeal joints. They are important muscles for gripping. For a child with weakness of the lumbrical muscles and poor handwriting, the problem is related to difficulty in maintaining adequate grip on the writing utensil. Grading of the activity would start with gripping a large utensil, such as tongs, then progressing to gripping of utensils of smaller diameter with the ultimate goal of gripping a pencil. Answer B is the only choice that deals with the gripping aspect of writing.

151. A, C, E: Scholarly activity goes hand in hand with evidence-based practice. Based on Boyer's approach to scholarship, scholarly activities should include discovery, integration, application, and teaching of knowledge. Attendance at the AOTA conference, participation in clinical research studies, and review of articles in the peer-reviewed *American Journal of Occupational Therapy* are all examples of scholarly activity. Interdisciplinary patient rounds are meetings to discuss the status

Copyright © Mometrix Media. You have been licensed one copy of this document for personal use only. Any other reproduction or redistribution is strictly prohibited. All rights reserved.
This content is provided for test preparation purposes only and does not imply an endorsement by Mometrix of any particular political, scientific, or religious point of view.

of specific patients by the rehabilitation team and are not considered to be scholarly activities. Annual infection control training is a mandatory training for facility-based health care providers. Although this training is based on research, to qualify as scholarly activity, the training would need to include activities such as the review of current research articles or participation in clinical research of infection control procedure. Last, blog postings, even those on the AOTA website, are not necessarily research based. Many times, blog postings include professional opinions that are not always based on evidence.

152. B,D,F: Based on the AOTA's therapy practice framework, a leisure activity is defined as "a nonobligatory activity that is intrinsically motivated and engaged in during discretionary time, that is, time not committed to obligatory occupations such as work, self-care, or sleep." The client should have the freedom of choice to choose a leisure activity that suits their needs. The leisure activity should give the person a sense of competence or accomplishment and intrinsic satisfaction. By definition, a leisure activity should not revolve around work or self-care. Suspension of reality is the freedom from the unnecessary constraints of reality and is a component of play activities, not leisure activities. For example, pretend play involves the suspension of reality.

153. C: Hand pain associated with rheumatoid arthritis can be treated with a paraffin bath. Acute injuries, especially with significant swelling, should be treated with cryotherapy, not heat. A recent surgical procedure would have a healing surgical wound. Use of heat would be contraindicated for this patient.

154. A: Children with Downs syndrome often present with atlantoaxial instability of the cervical spine. Therefore, any activities that could potentially cause a direct downward force on the cervical spine should be avoided, including tumbling activities.

155. B: Osteoporosis, autonomic dysreflexia, spasticity, and heterotopic ossification are all potential complications of a spinal cord injury. However, the symptoms of swelling, warmth, and decreased range of motion occurring between 1 and 4 months after a spinal cord injury are associated with heterotopic ossification.

156. A: To ascend a curb independently, a front approach is utilized (Answer A). Answer B describes the backward approach to ascending a curb that is only appropriate when an assistant is helping to move the wheelchair up the curb. To perform a partial wheelie to ascend the curb, the anti-tippers should be in the up position, not the down position. Therefore, Answer C is incorrect.

157. C: In this case scenario, the patient will require a communication device only while on the respirator. For temporary use to communicate basic needs, the low-technology communication board would be the most appropriate form of assistive technology. The speech-generating device and virtual keyboard with a pointer system are more advanced technology that are utilized by clients with long-term needs.

158. A: Using a light-colored plate with a dark border will increase the contrast and make the plate easier for the patient with low vision to see. On the other hand, placing a dark plate on a dark background will decrease the contrast, making it more difficult to see the plate. Placing any object on a patterned background will camouflage the object. Solid-colored backgrounds are much better to use as a background surface.

159. C: A patient with an L4 ASIA A spinal cord injury has a complete spinal cord injury, resulting in complete paralysis of bilateral LEs. The patient would utilize a strap to connect the leg rests to prevent the legs from moving posteriorly. For a patient with complete bilateral lower extremity paralysis, the strap is better at maintaining the positioning of the legs than heel loops, especially for

Copyright © Mometrix Media. You have been licensed one copy of this document for personal use only. Any other reproduction or redistribution is strictly prohibited. All rights reserved.
This content is provided for test preparation purposes only and does not imply an endorsement by Mometrix of any particular political, scientific, or religious point of view.

spastic paralysis. A patient with a C3 ASIA B spinal cord injury will not have any motor function below the neurological level. This patient would not be appropriate for a manual wheelchair. Both a transfemoral amputee and a transtibial amputee would utilize an amputee board or swing-away amputee attachment to position the residual limb. The leg rest on the involved side is not needed. If the patient has a prosthesis, then the leg rest with heel straps would be most appropriate.

160. A: If the wheelchair is too wide for a patient, the distance between the armrests will be increased, resulting in a less efficient push-up through the arms during transfers. Excessive pressure on the greater trochanters occurs when the wheelchair seat width is too narrow. The inability to position the legs under a table occurs when the seat height is too high.

161. C, E, F: There are three different approaches to modifying tasks to compensate for impairments. Tasks can be modified by changing the task method, changing the task objects, and changing the task environment. In this case scenario, the COTA is changing the task method. Sponge bathing at the sink instead of showering is an example of modifying the method. Likewise, dressing the affected side first and tying shoes with the one-handed approach are examples of modifying the task method. Using modified equipment such as a button hook or modified cutting board are examples of modification to the task object. The installation of a grab bar is an example of a modification to the task environment.

162. D: Answers A and D are examples of grading activities from easy to hard. Answers B and C are examples of modifications of task objects. Progressing from stirring a liquid to stirring cookie batter would increase the resistance level, making it harder to stir. Thus, this would be an appropriate activity for functional strengthening of the upper extremity. Progressing from an activity sitting to the same activity standing would be appropriate to improve balance and stability but not to improve functional strength of the upper extremity.

163. B: Typically, a patient will utilize ipsilateral scapular elevation and/or contralateral trunk flexion to compensate for weakness in the supraspinatus muscle, which initiates shoulder abduction. Shoulder external rotation will occur during end-range shoulder abduction as part of a combined motion pattern, not a substitution pattern. Shoulder internal rotation would not be a substitution pattern for shoulder abduction.

164. A, B, D: A person with a multiple-level cervical fusion will have limited cervical range of motion, resulting in difficulty turning the head while driving. A back-up camera and wide-angle mirrors would be appropriate to compensate for limited cervical range of motion. A person wearing a lower extremity prosthesis will not be able to feel the brake and gas pedals; therefore, hand controls for acceleration and braking would be necessary. A foot pedal extension would not be necessary as this person would not be safe to use foot pedals for braking or accelerating. The case scenario indicates that the person is ambulatory and does not indicate that the person has difficulty with transfers. Therefore, the transfer board would not be indicated.

165. A, C, F: To increase the complexity of an activity and make it more challenging, the COTA could increase the number of steps in the activity. Decreasing the number of steps would make the activity easier. Decreasing the frequency of verbal cues would make the activity more challenging because the patient would have to recall and problem-solve more when the verbal cues are decreased. Decreasing the amount of physical assistance that the COTA provides to the patient would require more physical exertion by the patient.

166. A, D, E: Impulsive behavior occurs when a patient acts before formulating a plan. Rather than waiting for instructions or considering the consequences, the impulsive patient will quickly take

Copyright © Mometrix Media. You have been licensed one copy of this document for personal use only. Any other reproduction or redistribution is strictly prohibited. All rights reserved.
This content is provided for test preparation purposes only and does not imply an endorsement by Mometrix of any particular political, scientific, or religious point of view.

action, often creating a safety risk. Behavioral intervention strategies to address impulsivity include step-by step written instructions, slow provision of verbal cues, and a calm, non-distracting environment. A group setting is distracting and should be avoided in the treatment of an impulsive patient. Allowing the patient to choose among activities may be appropriate for frustrated patients who benefit from feeling in control but will not curb impulsive behavior. Avoidance of repetitive tasks is appropriate for perseverative patients but is not an appropriate strategy for an impulsive patient.

167. B, D, E: Patients with a left-sided cerebrovascular accident will present with right hemiplegia and right visual field cuts. They will also have problems with language, time concepts, and analytical thinking. A right-sided cerebrovascular accident will present with left hemiplegia and left visual field cuts as well as impulsivity and impaired spatial orientation.

168. B, C, E: A patient with a right-sided cerebrovascular accident will present with involvement of the left side of the body. Therefore, this patient will not be able to utilize the left upper extremity and left lower extremity for wheelchair propulsion. The patient will not be able to use the right lower extremity to propel the wheelchair due to the right transfemoral amputation. Because the patient has full functioning only of the right upper extremity, a one-arm drive would be appropriate to allow the patient to propel a manual wheelchair. A lightweight wheelchair will be easier to propel and require less energy expenditure. Brake extenders will allow the patient to reach across the body with the right arm to lock the left brake. Elevating leg rests would not be necessary for a patient with left lower extremity paralysis who wears a prosthesis on the right side. Projection rims are designed to help people with decreased grip strength to propel the wheelchair. These are most often utilized by patients with lower cervical spinal cord injuries. Quick release wheels allow a person to take the wheels off the frame quickly. These are most typically utilized by patients who have good upper body strength and who disassemble their rigid-frame wheelchairs to fit them in a car.

169. C: Deep inhalation occurs through the nose. Slow exhalation through pursed lips should take twice as long as the inhalation.

170. B: Dyspnea control postures are positions that make breathing easier and allow for use of accessory muscles for breathing. Postures utilize a forward lean that incorporates a moderate amount of forward bending. Of all the answer choices, only Answers B and D incorporate forward leaning. Answer D does not provide sufficient forward bending and also places the patient in a position that could compress the axillary nerves. Answer B provides a moderate amount of forward bending and allows the patient to lean through the forearms on the shopping cart.

171. B, C, D: The frame of reference for the group activity should be client based, not based on scholarly research. A client-centered group activity should focus on the person–environment–occupation relationship and the development of a therapeutic relationship with the group members through the therapeutic use of self. Group activities should be flexible and individualized, not structured and generalized. The group leader should create an environment that facilitates change but should not actively attempt to promote change in the behavior of the group members.

172. C, E, F: The maximum protection phase is the first rehabilitation stage after surgery and usually lasts for 4 weeks, depending on the surgeon's protocol. Goals of this phase focus on surgical wound care; control of edema, pain, and inflammation; and early range-of-motion (ROM) exercises. The early ROM exercises should include AROM to the shoulder, wrist, and hand as well as self-assisted elbow flexion or extension and self-assisted forearm pronation or supination with the elbow partially flexed. Strengthening of the elbow through resisted isometrics does not occur

Copyright © Mometrix Media. You have been licensed one copy of this document for personal use only. Any other reproduction or redistribution is strictly prohibited. All rights reserved.
This content is provided for test preparation purposes only and does not imply an endorsement by Mometrix of any particular political, scientific, or religious point of view.

during this first stage of rehab. Strengthening of the shoulder utilizing cuff weights distal to the elbow would be contraindicated during this stage of rehabilitation. The placement of the cuff weights below the elbow would create stress through the elbow joint and would not be appropriate for a postoperative patient. End-range AROM elbow flexion is not appropriate during this stage of rehabilitation and would place stress on the surgical incision.

173. B: The curved utensils with enlarged handles, universal cuff for utensils, and the rocker knife would all be appropriate adaptive equipment for a patient with rheumatoid arthritis. However, due to the severe ulnar drift, the patient would have significant difficulty with any gripping activity. Therefore, the most appropriate utensil would be the universal cuff utensil holder.

174. A: All of the answer choices are adaptive cups; however, only the flow-control cup will affect the act of swallowing. The weighted bottom cup and the two-handled cup are used to make it easier to lift the cup to the mouth.

175. C, D, E: The somatosensory system provides information about the body's position in relationship to the supporting surface as well as the relationship of one body part to another. The visual system provides information relative to the position of the head relative to the environment, gaze stabilization, and the direction and speed of head movements. Changing the supporting surface to foam or an incline board will challenge the somatosensory system. Likewise, narrowing the base of support will also challenge the somatosensory system. Closing the eyes, wearing prism glasses, and moving the head and eyes will challenge the visual system.

176. C: Open-chain exercises are exercises in which the distal segment of the limb moves in space without simultaneous motion in adjacent joints. Open-chain exercises utilize non-weight-bearing positions of the involved extremity. Closed-chain exercises occur when the distal segment is fixed, and the proximal segments are moving. Closed-chain exercises utilize weight-bearing positions of the involved extremity. Wall push-ups involve weight-bearing through the hand on the wall with movement occurring through the proximal upper extremity joints. The exercises for bicep curls, lateral pulldowns, and grip strengthening are all open-chain exercises.

177. A: A transcutaneous electrical nerve stimulation (TENS) unit is an appropriate treatment to manage acute, postoperative, and chronic pain. NMES is utilized for muscle re-education. Superficial and deep heat are not appropriate in the treatment of acute conditions. Therefore, hydrocollator packs and continuous ultrasound would not be utilized to treat acute postoperative pain.

178. C: The standing, walking, and sitting hip (SWASH) orthosis is designed to promote hip abduction and reduce hip adductor tone, thereby improving stability in the seated position. The hip-knee-ankle-foot orthosis (HKAFO) provides stability to the hip, knee, ankle, and foot. The HKAFO does not promote sitting balance and is not appropriate for people with spasticity. Both the Milwaukee brace and the Wilmington brace are spinal orthoses and will not have any effect on the lower extremities.

179. D: The Stroop effect is an exercise to promote alternating attention by first having the client read the printed words then ignore the words and state the colors that the words are written in.

180. A: A buddy splint is a strap that is wrapped around two fingers and can be used to promote movement in a stiff finger by moving the other finger. Buddy splints are not designed to block motion or to immobilize a joint.

181. A, B, D: A return-to-work program focuses on getting the injured worker back to work as soon as possible. Modifications are made to the specific job tasks, work environment, and other areas

Copyright © Mometrix Media. You have been licensed one copy of this document for personal use only. Any other reproduction or redistribution is strictly prohibited. All rights reserved.
This content is provided for test preparation purposes only and does not imply an endorsement by Mometrix of any particular political, scientific, or religious point of view.

such as productivity requirements and work hours. In this case scenario, the worker sits at a desk for the majority of the day as a data entry clerk. Therefore, the ergonomic changes to the workstation are appropriate for this person, but the requirement of a second person for lifting more than 50 pounds and the limitation of prolonged standing do not match this person's job requirements. Starting back to work with reduced hours and reduced productivity requirements are appropriate to ease him or her back into the normal work routine. Because, the goal of a return-to-work program is for return to work as soon as possible, the injured worker would be allowed more rest breaks than the state requirements to provide time for symptom management, such as stretching and changing position.

182. C: For a patient whose primary limiting factor is fatigue, the most appropriate medical equipment for independent community mobility would be a motorized scooter. Lower-extremity fatigue would be a factor with use of either the rolling walker or the rollator. Upper-extremity fatigue would be a factor with use of the manual wheelchair.

183. A, B, E: Electrical stimulation should not be performed over the anterior cervical area due to the location of the vagus nerve, phrenic nerve, and carotid sinuses. Electrical stimulation causes increased blood flow; therefore, treatment should not be performed over cancerous areas because the increased circulation can potentially cause the tumors to spread. Similarly, osteomyelitis is a localized infection, and electrical stimulation should not be performed in the area of the infection. Open wounds can be treated with electrical stimulation and are not contraindications. However, certain precautions should be used in areas with open wounds or fragile skin. Pain can be effectively managed with electrical stimulation, such as transcutaneous electrical nerve stimulation (TENS); therefore, complex regional pain syndrome would not be a contraindication.

184. B, D, F: Continuous passive motion (CPM) is often used to gain range of motion after an orthopedic surgery such as a total knee replacement, which is performed on an arthritic knee. Therefore, osteoarthritis, recent orthopedic surgery, and a postsurgical wound would not be contraindications to use of a CPM machine. A postsurgical wound would be a precaution as care is needed not to position straps over the wound or to pull on the wound edges. Unstable fractures should not be treated with CPM as this could cause bone displacement and bone union delay. Patients with spasticity in the affected area should not receive CPM treatment because the CPM could trigger an increase in spasticity. CPM should not be administered in the area of an uncontrolled local infection as this could delay healing.

185. A, D, F: An acute, localized dermatological infection is a contraindication to use an intermittent compression pump because contact with the stockinette and/or compression sleeve and perspiration could cause the infection to spread. Acute pulmonary edema and congestive heart failure are contraindications to the use of an intermittent compression pump because the use of the pump places increased stress on the already compromised heart and lungs. Venous edema, venous leg ulcer, and lymphedema are all conditions that can be treated with an intermittent compression pump.

186. B: Inflation pressure is the maximum amount of pressure achieved during the inflation period of intermittent compression. Inflation pressure should not exceed diastolic pressure minus 10 mm Hg. Pressures higher than diastolic blood pressure have the potential to collapse blood vessels.

187. B: Pusher syndrome occurs in some patients after a stroke. Patients with pusher syndrome will lean heavily toward the hemiplegic side but will feel like they are standing in midline. Standing activities that utilize a mirror for feedback are appropriate to help the patient with pusher syndrome discover midline. Attempting to passively move the patient into a position will increase

Copyright © Mometrix Media. You have been licensed one copy of this document for personal use only. Any other reproduction or redistribution is strictly prohibited. All rights reserved.
This content is provided for test preparation purposes only and does not imply an endorsement by Mometrix of any particular political, scientific, or religious point of view.

the pushing toward the hemiplegic side. Lowering, not raising, the height of the assistive device on the uninvolved side can help the patient shift weight toward the uninvolved side, thus reducing the lean toward the hemiplegic side.

188. C: The cold snack of crackers and lunchmeat would be appropriate as an initial trial of meal preparation. Tasks will be graded to involve more challenges of cognition and safety, such as timed cooking activities and managing hot foods.

189. A: All of the answer choices are appropriate means of grading an activity; however, the only answer choice that has a social component is Answer A. Adding a level of competition to the activity will foster a social relationship between the patient and his or her competitor(s). Adding a level of frustration to the activity is a means of grading emotional factors. Changing the memory demands is a means of grading cognitive factors. Requiring the patient to initiate the activity is a means of grading temporal context.

190. C, D, F: Rewarding positive behavior, making activities fun, and having students earn the privilege of group participation are all strategies to promote good group dynamics in school-age children. Although it is appropriate to have a quiet area for the overstimulated student to take a rest in an area away from the group, a time-out chair in the hallway is not appropriate. Likewise, having behavioral rules is appropriate for the functioning of the group; however, the students should take an active role in establishing the rules and should stick with broad versus specific rules. Last, the group leader should pick their battles when addressing disruptive behavior and not address all behaviors equally. Minor misbehaviors may, in some cases, be best ignored.

191. C: The most appropriate prosthetic knee for a patient with cognitive deficits is the locking knee because it is the simplest to operate and the most stable. The locking knee promotes safety because it remains locked through all phases of gait and will not buckle. The weight-activated knee is capable of flexing during swing phase and will temporarily lock into knee extension during heel strike. The knee unit could buckle if the patient does not attain full knee extension upon heel strike. The microprocessor knee utilizes computerized components to control all aspects of gait and would be too complicated for a patient with cognitive deficits to operate.

192. A: A suction suspension utilizes a thin sock to don the socket, then the sock is pulled out of the socket through a valve to allow for an airtight seal to form between the skin and the socket.

193. B, E, F: Bathing should be performed with warm water. The residual limb should be dried thoroughly with a towel to eliminate moisture as this could lead to the development of an infection. Because bathing will soften the skin and cause slight edema, bathing should be performed in the evening after the patient is done using the prosthesis for the day. The use of rubbing alcohol and lotions should be avoided. Patients should be taught to examine their residual limb for signs of skin breakdown. Use of a long-handled mirror allows the patient to examine all aspects of the limb.

194. A, C, F: Removable rigid dressings, residual limb wrapping techniques, and shrinkers are utilized to provide compression to the residual limb to control edema. Placing a pillow under the knee of a patient with a transtibial amputation does not create adequate elevation to be an effective treatment for edema. It is also contraindicated because it can contribute to a knee flexion contracture. Transcutaneous electrical nerve stimulation (TENS) is an appropriate treatment for pain but not edema. Friction massage will mobilize scar tissue and desensitize the tissue but will not reduce edema.

195. D: Rhythmic stabilization exercises are isometric exercises that are performed against multidirectional, manual resistance to promote co-contraction of the agonist and antagonist

Copyright © Mometrix Media. You have been licensed one copy of this document for personal use only. Any other reproduction or redistribution is strictly prohibited. All rights reserved.
This content is provided for test preparation purposes only and does not imply an endorsement by Mometrix of any particular political, scientific, or religious point of view.

muscles and, thereby, promote postural stability. Multiple-angle isometric exercises are isometric exercises that are performed at joint positions within the available range of motion. Multiple-angle isometric exercises are utilized to improve strength throughout the range of motion when dynamic resistive exercises would be painful or contraindicated. Slow reversal hold exercises involve dynamic concentric contraction of a stronger agonist pattern, then dynamic concentric contraction of the weaker antagonist pattern, followed by an isometric hold at the end of the range. This exercise promotes dynamic stability of proximal joints of the extremities. The goal of rhythmic initiation is to promote the patient's ability to initiate a movement pattern. Rhythmic initiation consists of passive techniques performed by the therapist to help the patient become familiar with components of a movement pattern, progressing to active-assisted and active movement through the movement pattern.

196. B, C, D: The Mendelsohn maneuver is a swallowing exercise to raise the larynx and open the esophagus. Therefore, the Mendelsohn maneuver is appropriate to treat reduced closure at the laryngeal entrance, reduced laryngeal excursion, and limited cricopharyngeal opening. Slow pharyngeal transit is treated with the Lee Silverman Voice Treatment. Reduced base of tongue movement is treated by techniques such as the effortful swallow, Masako maneuver, and super-supraglottic swallow.

197. B, D, E: Ergonomic guidelines promote work postures that reduce the risk for injury while maximizing work performance. Computer workstations should be arranged with the computer screen approximately 20 inches from the eyes. The monitor should be positioned so the top border of the screen falls slightly below eye level. Shoulders should be relaxed at the sides of the body.

198. A: To stretch a muscle, the muscle's position should be the opposite of its position of contraction. Because the wrist extensors extend the wrist with radial deviation, the position of stretch must involve wrist flexion and ulnar deviation.

199. D, E, F: Gravity-eliminated or gravity-decreased positions are utilized for strengthening muscles that are graded poor to fair because these muscles are not strong enough to move against gravity. Equipment that reduces the effects of gravity or reduces friction is utilized at this stage of rehabilitation. Powder boards, skateboards, and suspension slings are examples of appropriate rehab equipment to be used by this patient. Resistive equipment such as a cable column, cuff weights, and TheraBand would not be appropriate at this stage.

200. C: Desensitization programs begin with tactile stimuli that are the least likely to produce a painful response from the patient then progress to more obtrusive stimuli. Fluidotherapy is less likely to elicit a pain reaction than constant pressure or a friction massage and therefore would be utilized before either of these treatments.

Copyright © Mometrix Media. You have been licensed one copy of this document for personal use only. Any other reproduction or redistribution is strictly prohibited. All rights reserved.
This content is provided for test preparation purposes only and does not imply an endorsement by Mometrix of any particular political, scientific, or religious point of view.

How to Overcome Test Anxiety

Just the thought of taking a test is enough to make most people a little nervous. A test is an important event that can have a long-term impact on your future, so it's important to take it seriously and it's natural to feel anxious about performing well. But just because anxiety is normal, that doesn't mean that it's helpful in test taking, or that you should simply accept it as part of your life. Anxiety can have a variety of effects. These effects can be mild, like making you feel slightly nervous, or severe, like blocking your ability to focus or remember even a simple detail.

If you experience test anxiety—whether severe or mild—it's important to know how to beat it. To discover this, first you need to understand what causes test anxiety.

Causes of Test Anxiety

While we often think of anxiety as an uncontrollable emotional state, it can actually be caused by simple, practical things. One of the most common causes of test anxiety is that a person does not feel adequately prepared for their test. This feeling can be the result of many different issues such as poor study habits or lack of organization, but the most common culprit is time management. Starting to study too late, failing to organize your study time to cover all of the material, or being distracted while you study will mean that you're not well prepared for the test. This may lead to cramming the night before, which will cause you to be physically and mentally exhausted for the test. Poor time management also contributes to feelings of stress, fear, and hopelessness as you realize you are not well prepared but don't know what to do about it.

Other times, test anxiety is not related to your preparation for the test but comes from unresolved fear. This may be a past failure on a test, or poor performance on tests in general. It may come from comparing yourself to others who seem to be performing better or from the stress of living up to expectations. Anxiety may be driven by fears of the future—how failure on this test would affect your educational and career goals. These fears are often completely irrational, but they can still negatively impact your test performance.

Elements of Test Anxiety

As mentioned earlier, test anxiety is considered to be an emotional state, but it has physical and mental components as well. Sometimes you may not even realize that you are suffering from test anxiety until you notice the physical symptoms. These can include trembling hands, rapid heartbeat, sweating, nausea, and tense muscles. Extreme anxiety may lead to fainting or vomiting. Obviously, any of these symptoms can have a negative impact on testing. It is important to recognize them as soon as they begin to occur so that you can address the problem before it damages your performance.

The mental components of test anxiety include trouble focusing and inability to remember learned information. During a test, your mind is on high alert, which can help you recall information and stay focused for an extended period of time. However, anxiety interferes with your mind's natural processes, causing you to blank out, even on the questions you know well. The strain of testing during anxiety makes it difficult to stay focused, especially on a test that may take several hours. Extreme anxiety can take a huge mental toll, making it difficult not only to recall test information but even to understand the test questions or pull your thoughts together.

Copyright © Mometrix Media. You have been licensed one copy of this document for personal use only. Any other reproduction or redistribution is strictly prohibited. All rights reserved.
This content is provided for test preparation purposes only and does not imply an endorsement by Mometrix of any particular political, scientific, or religious point of view.

Effects of Test Anxiety

Test anxiety is like a disease—if left untreated, it will get progressively worse. Anxiety leads to poor performance, and this reinforces the feelings of fear and failure, which in turn lead to poor performances on subsequent tests. It can grow from a mild nervousness to a crippling condition. If allowed to progress, test anxiety can have a big impact on your schooling, and consequently on your future.

Test anxiety can spread to other parts of your life. Anxiety on tests can become anxiety in any stressful situation, and blanking on a test can turn into panicking in a job situation. But fortunately, you don't have to let anxiety rule your testing and determine your grades. There are a number of relatively simple steps you can take to move past anxiety and function normally on a test and in the rest of life.

Physical Steps for Beating Test Anxiety

While test anxiety is a serious problem, the good news is that it can be overcome. It doesn't have to control your ability to think and remember information. While it may take time, you can begin taking steps today to beat anxiety.

Just as your first hint that you may be struggling with anxiety comes from the physical symptoms, the first step to treating it is also physical. Rest is crucial for having a clear, strong mind. If you are tired, it is much easier to give in to anxiety. But if you establish good sleep habits, your body and mind will be ready to perform optimally, without the strain of exhaustion. Additionally, sleeping well helps you to retain information better, so you're more likely to recall the answers when you see the test questions.

Getting good sleep means more than going to bed on time. It's important to allow your brain time to relax. Take study breaks from time to time so it doesn't get overworked, and don't study right before bed. Take time to rest your mind before trying to rest your body, or you may find it difficult to fall asleep.

Along with sleep, other aspects of physical health are important in preparing for a test. Good nutrition is vital for good brain function. Sugary foods and drinks may give a burst of energy but this burst is followed by a crash, both physically and emotionally. Instead, fuel your body with protein and vitamin-rich foods.

Also, drink plenty of water. Dehydration can lead to headaches and exhaustion, especially if your brain is already under stress from the rigors of the test. Particularly if your test is a long one, drink water during the breaks. And if possible, take an energy-boosting snack to eat between sections.

Along with sleep and diet, a third important part of physical health is exercise. Maintaining a steady workout schedule is helpful, but even taking 5-minute study breaks to walk can help get your blood pumping faster and clear your head. Exercise also releases endorphins, which contribute to a positive feeling and can help combat test anxiety.

When you nurture your physical health, you are also contributing to your mental health. If your body is healthy, your mind is much more likely to be healthy as well. So take time to rest, nourish your body with healthy food and water, and get moving as much as possible. Taking these physical steps will make you stronger and more able to take the mental steps necessary to overcome test anxiety.

Copyright © Mometrix Media. You have been licensed one copy of this document for personal use only. Any other reproduction or redistribution is strictly prohibited. All rights reserved.
This content is provided for test preparation purposes only and does not imply an endorsement by Mometrix of any particular political, scientific, or religious point of view.

Mental Steps for Beating Test Anxiety

Working on the mental side of test anxiety can be more challenging, but as with the physical side, there are clear steps you can take to overcome it. As mentioned earlier, test anxiety often stems from lack of preparation, so the obvious solution is to prepare for the test. Effective studying may be the most important weapon you have for beating test anxiety, but you can and should employ several other mental tools to combat fear.

First, boost your confidence by reminding yourself of past success—tests or projects that you aced. If you're putting as much effort into preparing for this test as you did for those, there's no reason you should expect to fail here. Work hard to prepare; then trust your preparation.

Second, surround yourself with encouraging people. It can be helpful to find a study group, but be sure that the people you're around will encourage a positive attitude. If you spend time with others who are anxious or cynical, this will only contribute to your own anxiety. Look for others who are motivated to study hard from a desire to succeed, not from a fear of failure.

Third, reward yourself. A test is physically and mentally tiring, even without anxiety, and it can be helpful to have something to look forward to. Plan an activity following the test, regardless of the outcome, such as going to a movie or getting ice cream.

When you are taking the test, if you find yourself beginning to feel anxious, remind yourself that you know the material. Visualize successfully completing the test. Then take a few deep, relaxing breaths and return to it. Work through the questions carefully but with confidence, knowing that you are capable of succeeding.

Developing a healthy mental approach to test taking will also aid in other areas of life. Test anxiety affects more than just the actual test—it can be damaging to your mental health and even contribute to depression. It's important to beat test anxiety before it becomes a problem for more than testing.

Study Strategy

Being prepared for the test is necessary to combat anxiety, but what does being prepared look like? You may study for hours on end and still not feel prepared. What you need is a strategy for test prep. The next few pages outline our recommended steps to help you plan out and conquer the challenge of preparation.

Step 1: Scope Out the Test

Learn everything you can about the format (multiple choice, essay, etc.) and what will be on the test. Gather any study materials, course outlines, or sample exams that may be available. Not only will this help you to prepare, but knowing what to expect can help to alleviate test anxiety.

Step 2: Map Out the Material

Look through the textbook or study guide and make note of how many chapters or sections it has. Then divide these over the time you have. For example, if a book has 15 chapters and you have five days to study, you need to cover three chapters each day. Even better, if you have the time, leave an extra day at the end for overall review after you have gone through the material in depth.

If time is limited, you may need to prioritize the material. Look through it and make note of which sections you think you already have a good grasp on, and which need review. While you are studying, skim quickly through the familiar sections and take more time on the challenging parts.

Copyright © Mometrix Media. You have been licensed one copy of this document for personal use only. Any other reproduction or redistribution is strictly prohibited. All rights reserved.
This content is provided for test preparation purposes only and does not imply an endorsement by Mometrix of any particular political, scientific, or religious point of view.

Write out your plan so you don't get lost as you go. Having a written plan also helps you feel more in control of the study, so anxiety is less likely to arise from feeling overwhelmed at the amount to cover.

Step 3: Gather Your Tools

Decide what study method works best for you. Do you prefer to highlight in the book as you study and then go back over the highlighted portions? Or do you type out notes of the important information? Or is it helpful to make flashcards that you can carry with you? Assemble the pens, index cards, highlighters, post-it notes, and any other materials you may need so you won't be distracted by getting up to find things while you study.

If you're having a hard time retaining the information or organizing your notes, experiment with different methods. For example, try color-coding by subject with colored pens, highlighters, or post-it notes. If you learn better by hearing, try recording yourself reading your notes so you can listen while in the car, working out, or simply sitting at your desk. Ask a friend to quiz you from your flashcards, or try teaching someone the material to solidify it in your mind.

Step 4: Create Your Environment

It's important to avoid distractions while you study. This includes both the obvious distractions like visitors and the subtle distractions like an uncomfortable chair (or a too-comfortable couch that makes you want to fall asleep). Set up the best study environment possible: good lighting and a comfortable work area. If background music helps you focus, you may want to turn it on, but otherwise keep the room quiet. If you are using a computer to take notes, be sure you don't have any other windows open, especially applications like social media, games, or anything else that could distract you. Silence your phone and turn off notifications. Be sure to keep water close by so you stay hydrated while you study (but avoid unhealthy drinks and snacks).

Also, take into account the best time of day to study. Are you freshest first thing in the morning? Try to set aside some time then to work through the material. Is your mind clearer in the afternoon or evening? Schedule your study session then. Another method is to study at the same time of day that you will take the test, so that your brain gets used to working on the material at that time and will be ready to focus at test time.

Step 5: Study!

Once you have done all the study preparation, it's time to settle into the actual studying. Sit down, take a few moments to settle your mind so you can focus, and begin to follow your study plan. Don't give in to distractions or let yourself procrastinate. This is your time to prepare so you'll be ready to fearlessly approach the test. Make the most of the time and stay focused.

Of course, you don't want to burn out. If you study too long you may find that you're not retaining the information very well. Take regular study breaks. For example, taking five minutes out of every hour to walk briskly, breathing deeply and swinging your arms, can help your mind stay fresh.

As you get to the end of each chapter or section, it's a good idea to do a quick review. Remind yourself of what you learned and work on any difficult parts. When you feel that you've mastered the material, move on to the next part. At the end of your study session, briefly skim through your notes again.

But while review is helpful, cramming last minute is NOT. If at all possible, work ahead so that you won't need to fit all your study into the last day. Cramming overloads your brain with more information than it can process and retain, and your tired mind may struggle to recall even

Copyright © Mometrix Media. You have been licensed one copy of this document for personal use only. Any other reproduction or redistribution is strictly prohibited. All rights reserved.
This content is provided for test preparation purposes only and does not imply an endorsement by Mometrix of any particular political, scientific, or religious point of view.

previously learned information when it is overwhelmed with last-minute study. Also, the urgent nature of cramming and the stress placed on your brain contribute to anxiety. You'll be more likely to go to the test feeling unprepared and having trouble thinking clearly.

So don't cram, and don't stay up late before the test, even just to review your notes at a leisurely pace. Your brain needs rest more than it needs to go over the information again. In fact, plan to finish your studies by noon or early afternoon the day before the test. Give your brain the rest of the day to relax or focus on other things, and get a good night's sleep. Then you will be fresh for the test and better able to recall what you've studied.

Step 6: Take a Practice Test

Many courses offer sample tests, either online or in the study materials. This is an excellent resource to check whether you have mastered the material, as well as to prepare for the test format and environment.

Check the test format ahead of time: the number of questions, the type (multiple choice, free response, etc.), and the time limit. Then create a plan for working through them. For example, if you have 30 minutes to take a 60-question test, your limit is 30 seconds per question. Spend less time on the questions you know well so that you can take more time on the difficult ones.

If you have time to take several practice tests, take the first one open book, with no time limit. Work through the questions at your own pace and make sure you fully understand them. Gradually work up to taking a test under test conditions: sit at a desk with all study materials put away and set a timer. Pace yourself to make sure you finish the test with time to spare and go back to check your answers if you have time.

After each test, check your answers. On the questions you missed, be sure you understand why you missed them. Did you misread the question (tests can use tricky wording)? Did you forget the information? Or was it something you hadn't learned? Go back and study any shaky areas that the practice tests reveal.

Taking these tests not only helps with your grade, but also aids in combating test anxiety. If you're already used to the test conditions, you're less likely to worry about it, and working through tests until you're scoring well gives you a confidence boost. Go through the practice tests until you feel comfortable, and then you can go into the test knowing that you're ready for it.

Test Tips

On test day, you should be confident, knowing that you've prepared well and are ready to answer the questions. But aside from preparation, there are several test day strategies you can employ to maximize your performance.

First, as stated before, get a good night's sleep the night before the test (and for several nights before that, if possible). Go into the test with a fresh, alert mind rather than staying up late to study.

Try not to change too much about your normal routine on the day of the test. It's important to eat a nutritious breakfast, but if you normally don't eat breakfast at all, consider eating just a protein bar. If you're a coffee drinker, go ahead and have your normal coffee. Just make sure you time it so that the caffeine doesn't wear off right in the middle of your test. Avoid sugary beverages, and drink enough water to stay hydrated but not so much that you need a restroom break 10 minutes into the

Copyright © Mometrix Media. You have been licensed one copy of this document for personal use only. Any other reproduction or redistribution is strictly prohibited. All rights reserved.
This content is provided for test preparation purposes only and does not imply an endorsement by Mometrix of any particular political, scientific, or religious point of view.

test. If your test isn't first thing in the morning, consider going for a walk or doing a light workout before the test to get your blood flowing.

Allow yourself enough time to get ready, and leave for the test with plenty of time to spare so you won't have the anxiety of scrambling to arrive in time. Another reason to be early is to select a good seat. It's helpful to sit away from doors and windows, which can be distracting. Find a good seat, get out your supplies, and settle your mind before the test begins.

When the test begins, start by going over the instructions carefully, even if you already know what to expect. Make sure you avoid any careless mistakes by following the directions.

Then begin working through the questions, pacing yourself as you've practiced. If you're not sure on an answer, don't spend too much time on it, and don't let it shake your confidence. Either skip it and come back later, or eliminate as many wrong answers as possible and guess among the remaining ones. Don't dwell on these questions as you continue—put them out of your mind and focus on what lies ahead.

Be sure to read all of the answer choices, even if you're sure the first one is the right answer. Sometimes you'll find a better one if you keep reading. But don't second-guess yourself if you do immediately know the answer. Your gut instinct is usually right. Don't let test anxiety rob you of the information you know.

If you have time at the end of the test (and if the test format allows), go back and review your answers. Be cautious about changing any, since your first instinct tends to be correct, but make sure you didn't misread any of the questions or accidentally mark the wrong answer choice. Look over any you skipped and make an educated guess.

At the end, leave the test feeling confident. You've done your best, so don't waste time worrying about your performance or wishing you could change anything. Instead, celebrate the successful completion of this test. And finally, use this test to learn how to deal with anxiety even better next time.

Review Video: Test Anxiety
Visit mometrix.com/academy and enter code: 100340

Important Qualification

Not all anxiety is created equal. If your test anxiety is causing major issues in your life beyond the classroom or testing center, or if you are experiencing troubling physical symptoms related to your anxiety, it may be a sign of a serious physiological or psychological condition. If this sounds like your situation, we strongly encourage you to seek professional help.

Copyright © Mometrix Media. You have been licensed one copy of this document for personal use only. Any other reproduction or redistribution is strictly prohibited. All rights reserved.
This content is provided for test preparation purposes only and does not imply an endorsement by Mometrix of any particular political, scientific, or religious point of view.

Online Resources

Due to our efforts to try to keep this book to a manageable length, we've created a link that will give you access to all of your online resources:

mometrix.com/resources719/ota

It's Your Moment, Let's Celebrate It!

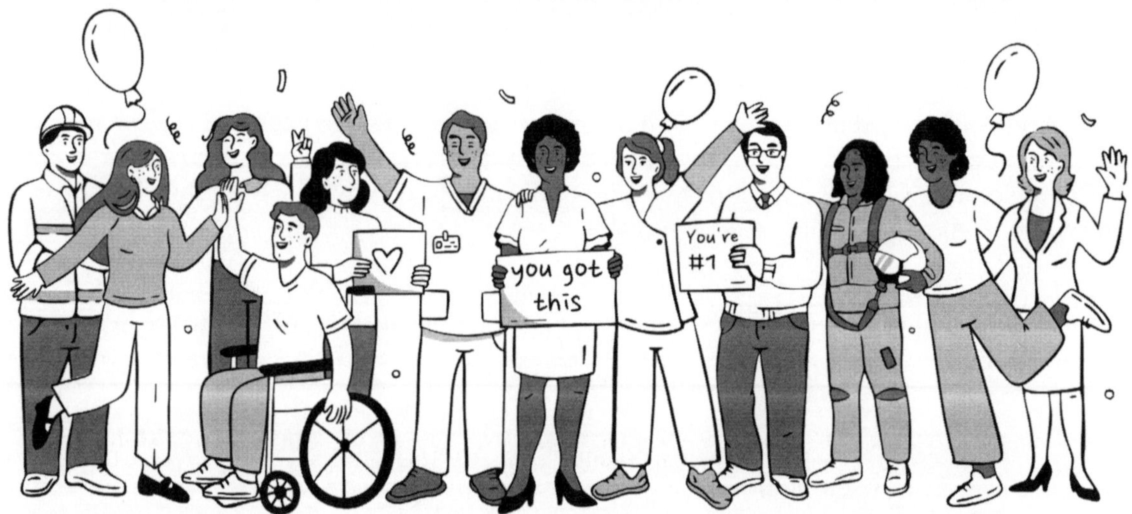

Share your story @mometrixtestpreparation

Copyright © Mometrix Media. You have been licensed one copy of this document for personal use only. Any other reproduction or redistribution is strictly prohibited. All rights reserved.
This content is provided for test preparation purposes only and does not imply an endorsement by Mometrix of any particular political, scientific, or religious point of view.